About the author

Brian Halvorsen is a member of the British Dental Association, the British Society for Nutritional Medicine, and is currently Treasurer of the British Dental Society for Clinical Nutrition. He combines a career as a dentist in general practice with freelance writing on dental health. He contributes the 'Dental Expert' column to *Here's Health*, along with other articles, and has been featured in interviews on both radio and television.

Since qualifying from Bristol University and the Royal College of Surgeons in 1974, he has developed a special interest in the relationship between dental health and general bodily well-being. He believes that dentists can play a far more important role in preventative medicine by providing health screening and dietary advice. His aim is to establish dentistry within the framework of an integrated health-care system.

Brian Halvorsen is a keen sportsman and gourmet, and lives with his wife and two sons (both of whom are free from fillings) in Buckinghamshire.

Acknowledgements

— First and foremost, to my lovely wife Lynda for her help and support with this book, and for our harmonious life together.
— To Ben and Adam, my sons, for giving a greater purpose and joy to our lives.
— To Chris Luttman, my secretary, for giving unselfishly of her time and enthusiasm.
— To Michael Moore for his unstinting help and friendship.
— To David Brooker, a fellow dentist, whose help and advice was greatly appreciated.
— And to Susan Fleming for her skill, professionalism and unfailing interest — simply a super person to work with.
— I thank you all.

THE NATURAL DENTIST

A holistic approach to the prevention of dental disease

Brian Halvorsen
with Susan Fleming

CENTURY ARROW
London Melbourne Auckland Johannesburg

To those who have
suffered through ignorance

A Century Arrow Book
Published by Arrow Books Limited
62–65 Chandos Place, London WC2N 4NW

An imprint of Century Hutchinson Ltd

London Melbourne Sydney Auckland
Johannesburg and agencies throughout
the world

First published 1986

Copyright © Brian Halvorsen 1986
Diagrams by Joy FitzSimmons

Photoset by Rowland Phototypesetting Ltd,
Bury St Edmunds, Suffolk

Printed and bound in Great Britain by
Hunt Barnard Printing Ltd, Aylesbury, Bucks.

ISBN 0 09 946720 8

Contents

Foreword

As more people are becoming aware of the overall importance of diet in relation to health, the thirst for sound, reliable information increases. Responsibility for good health lies in the hands of each one of us, but we also need a measure of common sense, and guidelines so that we can decide the best way of looking after ourselves. *The Natural Dentist* is an excellent source of information about how to look after teeth, and it is presented in an interesting and factual way. By following the recommendations in this book, the health of our teeth and those of our children will be greatly helped. Preventative dental care is well covered as is how to deal with certain existing problems of teeth and gums. Prevention of these problems is becoming more and more desirable as the cost of dental treatment increases, and the explanations here of how poor dental health occurs are particularly interesting – and from which I personally learned a lot. I am sure, too, that many parents will be interested to learn by reading this book how best to educate their children into correct dietary habits, and how and when to clean their teeth.

This book is a timely first in this country and should help a lot of people avoid much of the pain and suffering that are so often a consequence of having poor teeth. Prevention is better than cure – it's cheaper too. This book should be read by anybody with a mouth!

Dr Stephen Davies
Physician and Chairman of the British Society
for Nutritional Medicine

Introduction

If, as a consequence of not washing our hands properly, they were to wither away, we should probably use soap and water rather more frequently than was entirely necessary. If our legs were to show a tendency to drop off when we ate the wrong foods, we would undoubtedly make sure that the right foods were totally predominant in our diet. Yet this is what is happening in our mouths: we are not cleaning them properly, we are not eating a good diet, and thus the vast majority of us appear to be choosing to become dental cripples!

Every day of my practising career as a dentist, I observe some form of dental disease, either tooth decay or gum disease, and both of these, I believe, are almost totally preventable. And because they are so *easily* preventable, the frustration of dentists like myself can be readily appreciated. The most minor lifestyle changes – like better cleaning and a more sensible daily diet – can reduce disease in the mouth to almost negligible levels, yet somewhere along the line the message has not got through, and is still not getting through. Teeth are vital in so many ways – eating and good appearance are but two – but a majority seem not to care. A mere 50 per cent of the population in this country actually visits the dentist regularly, and dental care came only twentieth in a recent survey of spending priorities. In fact, in some parts of the country, it's accepted that you're lucky if you've still got your teeth after twenty-one; often it's not a case of saving up for the house deposit or a new car, but for the first set of full dentures!

This lemming-like attitude amazes and saddens me. When I – and indeed most dentists – tell patients how they can prevent dental disease, they often remark sarcastically: 'Well, if I do everything you tell me, you're going to do yourself out of a job.' It's touching, but somewhat ironic, that they should be worried about my well-being – my financial well-being in particular – to the detriment of their own health and that of their families. It could almost appear that they're trying, by ignoring their teeth, to keep dentists in business! And indeed business there always will be for dentists. Even if we do manage to eradicate dental disease totally – an ambition that is realizable, but a fairly long way off as yet – there still remains the management aspect of teeth and jaws: growth, development and appearance, major considerations upon which we cannot at the moment spend the time we would like.

The fact that dentists are, arguably, the most feared profession- al members of our society, may have something to do with this reluctance on the part of the public. 'I'd rather have a baby than have a tooth filled' is a common expression heard by the dentist – often from large muscle-bound men who are reduced to lumps of jelly on seeing a local anaesthetic needle or hearing the noise of the high-speed drill. An enormous number of phobias are built up around visiting the dentist, and certainly an image still persists of the dentist as driller-filler. But by those small lifestyle changes mentioned already, visiting the dentist could be much less trau- matic than it now is: by preventing the disease developing, the treatment which is most feared will, in the majority of cases, simply not be required.

And this is where the holistic or natural dentist comes in. The holistic practitioner – of whatever specilization – looks at the individual as a whole person. Each part of the body is seen in relationship to the rest of the body, and any diagnosis or treat- ment is seen in terms of the body as a whole, and how it will benefit the patient both physically and mentally. No part of the body is studied in isolation: a far cry from modern specialized dental training, during which many dentists, sadly, learn to look upon their patients as mere mouths on legs. And by relating disease in the mouth to an imbalance in the body in general, by using the mouth as a barometer of the health of the whole patient (and vice versa), the holistic or natural dentist is enabled to aspire to a much wider disease-prevention role in society.

It is nutrition that is his primary concern, for there is no doubt that it is correct nutrition that governs dental health. If nutrition and dentistry seem to be unlikely bedfellows, just consider the sugar question. The antipathy of dentists towards sugar in its more obvious confectionary forms is well known, and cutting out all sugar is a very good first step towards an improved dental health. But the refined and processed foods so prevalent today are bad for bodily as well as dental health, a finding graphically illustrated by the researches of an American dentist as long ago as the 1930s. Dr Weston Price studied numerous isolated peoples still living on natural diets, far from the influences of western civilization. Before they encountered modern foodstuffs such as white flours and sugars, they were healthy, happy and dentally very fit with wide jaws, wide dental arches and little tooth decay: within a generation, however, the situation had drastically changed, and the peoples – without exception – had altered behaviourally and physically, displaying tooth decay, narrow dental arches and poor skeletal structures in general. The book Dr Price published – *Nutrition and Physical Degeneration* – is full of before and after pictures which provide spectacular confirmation that nutrition has *everything* to do with dental health. That this is still being ignored to a large extent by doctors and dentists is alarming, to say the least.

Natural dentists will go even further than this, believing that gum disease and mouth ulcers, say, are also nutritionally based. Gum disease, for instance, is a case in point: if the body is poorly supplied nutritionally so that digestive problems ensue or organs are affected, then the mouth tissue too could similarly react – for the blood that flows to the gums is exactly the same blood that pumps through the heart and down to the toes. In the same way, the natural or holistic dentist is anxious about other substances the body ingests: fluoride and mercury are major concerns of many at the moment. Both are highly toxic, and yet they are widely used by dentists. Mass fluoridation of water supplies, for instance, is far removed from the individual diagnosis and treatment which is the aim of holistic dentists – and which should be the aim of all medical practitioners.

Dentists are in a unique position in our modern-day society. They have a wide knowledge of the disciplines of general medicine (although obviously not to the same degree as their medical colleagues), and they have a highly specialized knowledge of the mouth and its related disorders. They also see their patients on a regular basis, and thus are uniquely qualified to act as reviewers of health, operating a sort of early-warning system. A doctor will see a patient only when that patient is unwell and requires his services; a dentist will see patients at, ideally, six-monthly intervals and may be – as has often happened – the first one to spot the signs of early disease: a nutritional deficiency or the inimitable symptoms of stress, of which the patient may not even be aware. Indeed more than a few unexplained persistent head and back aches have been diagnosed and treated successfully by dentists investigating the TMJ syndrome, a malfunction of the jaw alignment.

Because the benefits of this medical screening are so potentially great, dentists can widen their scope and play a much more positive role in society's health. If they succeed in re-educating the public dentally, they will be more free to concentrate on health counselling, advising on the growth and development of their new patients from as early as the pre-conceptual stage, and this can ensure the physical and dental health of the generations to come.

Brian Halvorsen
March 1986

CHAPTER ONE

The History of Dentistry

The history of dentistry is interlaced with archaeology, diet, inventiveness (sometimes magnificently creative, sometimes quite horrific), pain, social customs and politics. And that history is long, for man, of course, has always had teeth – as well as, for the most part, tooth decay and gum disease. That we are still suffering from these same diseases centuries later, after all the advances in scientific knowledge, is amazing to me in my capacity as both a conventional and natural dentist: sugar, for instance, was recognized early as a cause of rotten teeth, but now we would appear to be eating more of it than ever before. And the fact that less than 50 per cent of the population go to the dentist regularly, that from surveys dental care has been shown to be twentieth in a list of spending priorities – *after* pet food – would seem to demonstrate that we have still not learned much about how important our teeth are.

In the Beginning

Teeth, made of one of the hardest natural substances, and certainly the most indestructible part of the human body, have proved vital clues in the search for our past. From skulls found in prehistoric sites around the world, and dating from many periods, the development of 'modern' man can be traced. As man evolved over hundreds of thousands of years, his physical appearance slowly altered: the most important change was in the shape of his skull, as the size of his brain increased; the second most important was in the shape of his jaw and in the size and variety of his teeth.

These latter, from present-day dental examinations, seem to have suffered little from tooth decay and gum disease.

Early ancestors of man had formidable canines or eye teeth, like today's baboons, but *Homo habilis* or 'handy man', who lived about 1¾ million years ago, had canines which were as small as our own today. The canines were fighting teeth, with which to threaten, to pierce, puncture and tear – think of the baboon's most aggressive gesture: throwing back his head and opening his mouth to display his teeth. The decrease in size of those canines in man probably went hand in hand with his development of the use of weapons and tools; now he was no longer reliant on physical attributes such as claws or teeth, but could make and design his own. Thus the necessity for those canines declined (although Dracula still makes a basically primitive use of his!), and this new-found ability, so amply demonstrated in teeth, was probably the key by which man ultimately gained mastery over all other species.

As brain size altered, so too did the shape of the jaw. The brain size of *Australopithecus* – who lived in Africa some 5 million years ago – was little larger than his ape cousin, and his jaws were prominent, with large and powerful teeth, in order to chew tough grains and raw meat. By the time of *Homo erectus*, who lived 4½ million years later, the brain had enlarged and the jaw had decreased in size, as had the teeth. *Homo erectus* used fire for warmth and probably for cooking too; as cooked meat is easier to chew than raw, the large flat molar or back teeth that earlier forms of man had developed were not as necessary. Those enormous teeth and massive jaws could thus be reduced in size to the more refined physical characteristics of modern man, and these have finally evolved over the last 30,000 years.

If tool-making was the key to man's dominance over the rest of the animal world, and the cooking of food heralded the beginnings of modern man, so cooking food could also be said perhaps to mark the beginnings of dental disease. Diet, I believe, is vital for healthy bodies and teeth, and it is at the core of this book. Primitive man, in a world entirely free of all our modern pollutants, lived a healthy – if relatively short and dangerous – life, and he ate a healthy diet of raw nuts, seeds, grasses, raw meats and fish. To complement this diet, and as a result of this diet, the dental arch – the wide curve of the teeth in both upper and lower jaws – was broad to allow room for the biting incisors and canines, and the grinding molars at the back. Foods that require active chewing were – and are – good for jaws and teeth. This spaciousness of the arch is still the prime requisite of a good jaw and healthy teeth today, and our smaller jaws often have to rely on orthodontics – which may necessitate the *removal* of teeth – to prevent crowding, and thus places between the teeth where the disease-carrying bacteria can flourish. So, as man began to cook his food – together with the processing of it (for processing of grains into flour, say, was also an early practice) – jaws decreased in size, teeth became more crowded, and mouth disease began.

The quality of this early food would have been much better, though, in terms of environment, vitamins and minerals etc., so the proportion of disease would have been small. And there were undeniably other factors in promoting tooth decay. Teeth of some Bronze Age skulls show decay which is probably the result of *too much* grinding, when pieces of bone, shell or grit, which inevitably attach to such basic foods, have worn down the surface of the teeth, creating holes into which bacteria could enter. However, if we were able to compare, say, 100 primitive men with a similar number of present-day men, the teeth of the former would undoubtedly be in much better condition.

Dentistry in Antiquity

There were no stone-age dentists because, on the whole, the teeth of stone-age man were in good condition. But very shortly afterwards – at least in terms of the history of man – ancient texts from all over the world begin to record diseases of the teeth and how to treat them.

A Sumerian clay tablet, 'The Legend of the Worm', dating from around 5000 BC, gives advice on how to rid the teeth of the small worms believed to cause toothache. This tooth-eating worm theory was to be associated with tooth decay for many centuries thereafter – and is really not so fanciful when we consider that many of the bacteria which cause decay are literally worm-shaped! Over 1,000 years later, a Sanskrit text had details on tooth surgery, and in the famous medical Ebers Papyrus – discovered in Egypt around 1862 and written in about 1500 BC (but copied, it is thought, from earlier papyri) – many ideas of treatment are listed, although no mention is made of any surgical or restorative procedures. And indeed, from the thousands of mummies examined over the years, the Ancient Egyptians – those of the upper classes anyway – would appear to have suffered greatly from dental disease: jaw bones and teeth show evidence of rampant gum disease and tooth decay and the resultant infection and shrinking of bone known as osteomyelitis. Although it is commonly believed that Ancient Egypt enjoyed the services of experts on teeth, who made dental appliances and fillings from gold, no proof of any dentistry has been found on any mummies. But if such 'dentists' had existed, they would surely have been employed by those entombed as mummies: if they were rich and important enough to face the afterlife thus, they would certainly have sought relief from the pain they so evidently suffered.

It was not until the time of the Etruscans – a people who lived in what is now Tuscany in Italy, and whose civilization stretched roughly from the eighth to the fourth centuries BC – that we have evidence of a high level of dentistry. Partial dentures – early dental bridges – have been found in tombs: bands of gold hold together the natural and artificial or substitute teeth (one such found was the tooth of a calf). No attempt was made to hide these golden bands – which covered a large proportion of the crown of the teeth – thus suggesting that they were worn with pride rather than in shame (rather like the gold teeth flashing proudly from many Mediterranean and African mouths today). The standard of technology was astoundingly high in comparison with what was to follow, in the 'Dark Ages', and it was not until the dawn of the nineteenth century that anything like the same standards were again achieved!

The Ancient Greeks and Romans suffered from tooth decay and gum disease as well. Hippocrates, the Greek 'Father of Medicine', recommended extraction when teeth were decayed or loose, although later writers, like Aristotle, were better dental anatomists. And the Roman medical writer, Aulus Cornelius Celsus, wrote, in about 25 BC to AD 35, of dental matters very near to the heart of this book: that poor teeth result from the processed or refined foods of civilization. In his *De Re Medicina* he advised the inhabitants of towns and cities to wash their mouths out well daily to prevent tooth decay; peasants did not need to bother, apparently, because of their simple and unrefined diet. Caius Plinius Secundus or Pliny the Elder (AD 23–79) echoed some of Celsus's ideas: 'A man's breath becomes infected by the bad quality of the food, by the bad state of his teeth and still more by old age.' This apparent scientific modernity is somewhat dashed by his renowned inability to distinguish between fact and fiction: he recorded a current belief that a frog tied to the jaws would make loose teeth firm!

In antiquity then, there was a variable degree of dental sophistication – but an unvarying amount of dental disease. It's difficult to generalize, of course, because the evidence such as it is points to a particular social class, an upper class who were buried in a more durable manner or whose ills were treated and recorded by their physicians. It does seem, however, that dentistry went hand in hand with civilization (as with any advancement of science, of course), and exhibited by the dental silence of the Dark Ages of the barbarians following the collapse of the Roman Empire. With civilization went a 'civilized' and thus refined diet; and with that went the diseases associated with diet, primarily dental disease.

Dentistry in the Middle Ages

The history of dentistry must make such a leap in time, as the science seemed to completely deteriorate in Europe. It was the Chinese – who used acupuncture to alleviate toothache as early as 2700 BC – and the Arabians who kept dental skills and research alive. Abulcasis (1050–1122) was regarded as the greatest Arabian surgeon of the Middle Ages, and his *De Chirurgia* remained a standard medical textbook for centuries thereafter. He set broken jaws with wire splints, improved extraction instruments, closed hare lips successfully – and was perhaps the first dental hygienist: in his book he illustrates many different dental scalers and described in detail the process of scaling (scraping off of tartar or calculus – which causes gum disease – from the teeth). It was not until 1308 in Britain that some semblance of organization attached itself to those who drew teeth: the barber-surgeons formed themselves into a guild. They were divided into two groups – those who practised barbery proper (phlebotomy or blood letting and tooth drawing: this is the meaning behind the colours of the traditional barber's pole – red for blood, white for teeth), and those who practised surgery. The guild remained active until 1745 after which the barbers separated to form a guild of their own.

Although the barber-surgeons did not become really common until the fifteenth century, work continued on the Continent. Guy de Chauliac (1309–1386), a French surgeon, wrote extensively on the teeth – although reiterating much of what Abulcasis had written 250 years earlier. He used soporific drugs to subdue pain, and in some manuscript copies of his great treatise, *Chirurgia Magna*, there appears for the first time the word 'dentista'. A century later, Giovanni Vigo, an Italian surgeon, advocated careful excavating and shaping of a tooth cavity before filling with gold leaf. Amboise Paré, a French surgeon, recorded transplantation of teeth, that dental decay is caused by worms (still continuing in the late sixteenth century), and that preventative measures such as filing the teeth, removing tartar and general mouth hygiene should be undertaken.

But for many years in Britain, only the barber-surgeons and their extraction methods were available, plus their main rivals, against whom the guild bitterly railed: the itinerant and unqualified tooth-drawers. These gentlemen, often wearing necklaces of teeth or hats decorated with teeth, would frequent markets and fairs, offering their services. Drums were beaten loudly and music played to drown the screams of the unfortunate sufferers. That they were many – and that their services were needed as well as dreaded – is evidenced by the prolific paintings and prints over the years of the common people suffering their attentions. The main instruments used were pliers or forceps, pelicans (with a claw to prise a tooth out), and elevators which had a tapering blade to elevate the roots of bad teeth.

The horrors of dental pain and tooth extraction are perhaps most clearly exemplified by the Virgin Queen Elizabeth I. She suffered severely from toothache from her childhood onwards, and according to a German visitor to her court had black teeth which he said was characteristic of the English in general because of their great love of sugar (and indeed sweetmeats, sweet puddings and cakes, and candied fruits etc., are the most famed aspect of English cuisine even today). It is recorded that Elizabeth, when once suffering badly from toothache, could only be persuaded to have the tooth out by Bishop Aylmer, who volunteered to have one of his drawn first to show that the pain wasn't as bad as she might expect. Greater love hath no man . . .

False teeth in England were rare at this time, and to fill out a mouth bereft of teeth Elizabeth would pad her jaws and cheeks with cloths in the interest of vanity. Many of her portraits – and indeed those of many other well-to-do people of the period – do show that teeth were few if not completely lacking. It's a particularly interesting exercise for dentists and dental students, but if you go to a gallery or to an historic house, look at the jaw position in portraits and how near the nose is to the chin. Many people in the portraits were obviously young and lacked teeth – and this is probably why none of the sitters are smiling!

Until the end of the seventeenth century in Britain, dental progress was negligible. There were attempts, though, at dentures for those who lacked teeth. Robert Herrick (1591–1674), a Cavalier poet (responsible for the immortal line 'Gather ye rosebuds while ye may'), wrote an ode 'Upon Glasco':

> Glasco had none, but now some teeth has got;
> Which though they furre, will neither ake nor rot.
> Six teeth he has, whereof twice two are known
> Made of a haft that was a mutton bone
> Which not for use, but meerly for the sight,
> He wears all day and drawes those teeth at night.

These dentures – often made, as suggested above, from animal bone, or carved from ivory for the very rich – conjure up a picture of a toothless nation, particularly the upper classes, who would be unable to eat or speak properly. More sophisticated dentures with which their wearer could eat or speak without clicking, movement or displacement – even shooting out – were not available until at least the beginning of the eighteenth century.

Work continued on the Continent at this time, however. In 1683, a Dutchman, Antony von Leeuwenhoek, described for the first time the presence of tiny animals in the debris around the human teeth, and opined that their numbers in one mouth probably exceeded the number of men in the country. He had taken some bacterial plaque from his own mouth and was the first person to look at it under a microscope. In 1700, the French College of Surgeons inaugurated a dental department and created the first examinations for dental practitioners. In 1712, one Nicol Facussi successfully implanted teeth obtained from corpses, and the practice of transplantation was to continue and expand over the next couple of centuries. Even 100 years later, after the Battle of Waterloo, hordes of scavengers raided the corpses of soldiers lying on the battlefield to extract their teeth for use in dentures.

The Beginnings of Modern Dentistry

In 1728, Pierre Fauchard (1678–1761), a French surgeon-dentist, published two volumes which made dental history: they were the first systematic attempt to record a complete picture of the practice of dentistry, and they brought about a distinction and separation of the practices of dentistry and surgery. From here onwards, the science itself, as well as treatment, prosthesis (the replacement by artificial limbs or teeth), and the making of dentures, crowns and bridges became more sophisticated.

In 1746 Pierre Mouton described the making of the gold shell crown for the first time; in 1757 the theory of worms in the teeth was disproved; in 1790 John Greenwood, an American dentist, invented a dental foot drill (he was also one of George Washington's dentists, and made him several teeth); and in 1771, John Hunter FRS, a surgeon and pathologist, published *The Natural History of the Human Teeth* which formed the basis for all modern texts on the jaw and teeth. He also experimented with transplanting of sound teeth. This barbaric practice became quite popular, and newspapers carried advertisements asking for natural human teeth. Poor unfortunates with good sound teeth, mainly children, would have them wrenched painfully from their mouths and these freshly extracted teeth would then promptly be implanted in the mouths of wealthy recipients. For this, the donor could be paid 2 guineas (a large amount then). Suitable slaves would also be used as donors, and they of course would be cheaper. And in 1775, Paul Revere, subject of Longfellow's poem, 'Paul Revere's Ride', was perhaps the first dentist to be called upon to identify a corpse – killed at the Battle of Bunker Hill – from its dental work.

At the very beginning of the nineteenth century, Joseph Fox was the first dental surgeon to be appointed to Guy's Hospital in London. By this time tooth filling had become more common, and he was advocating a mixture of bismuth, lead and tin. This was presumably as dangerous as the mercury which began to be used a few years later, cropping up again in 1826 when a French dentist used a filling amalgam of filings of silver 5-franc pieces mixed with mercury. When, in 1833, the Crawcour brothers introduced a similar amalgam to America, their methods were the cause of the 'amalgam war' of about 1835–1850, when the American Dental Association banned the use of amalgam.

In 1844, Horace Wells, a Connecticut dentist, demonstrated the anaesthetic properties for dentistry of nitrous oxide, laughing gas, and thereafter a new era in tooth pulling began. In the same year plaster of Paris was introduced for taking impressions of the teeth, another leap forward for those who had to wear ill-fitting dentures (measured up till then with compasses and, if they were lucky, wax). A few years later, Edwin Truman, Queen Victoria's dentist, introduced gutta percha – a latex gum derived from Malaysian trees – as the basis for artificial dentures (it was he who also coated the Atlantic cable with gutta percha, thus protecting it from the corrosion of sea water: it was also used in golfballs and chewing gum!). In 1848 Thomas Evans of Paris used vulcanite as a base for artificial dentures (a hard material made by heating rubber with sulphur); he made one such denture for Charles Goodyear Senior in 1854. A few years later Charles Goodyear Junior patented the use of caoutchouc or rubber as a base for artificial dentures, and the Goodyear tyre company received thereafter a royalty on every denture sold!

In 1891, the 'grand old man in dentistry', Green Vardiman Black (1836–1915) of Chicago, began the process of preventative dentistry proper. It was he who standardized cavity preparation – dentists still know Black's cavity today – and his researches revolutionized the use of amalgam fillings. With the dawning of the twentieth century, medicine and dentistry entered a new era following the development of significant scientific discoveries. Nearly 100 years have elapsed since one of the first films – that of a jaw and teeth – was developed from the use of X-rays. At about the same time the first local anaesthetics were being used, a very potent mixture of cocaine and morphine. Equipment and techniques used in the latter part of the century would certainly be recognized by today's dentists.

Dentistry as a Profession

In the seventeenth and eighteenth centuries, there was no real profession of dentistry, but as science improved, there was a divide. Some dentists became very skilful, studying anatomy of jaws and teeth, performing skilful operations and using sophisticated instruments. There were also those who were unskilled and unqualified: these 'dentists' got their work through advertising at fairgrounds etc. In 1839, the birth of organized dentistry occurred, with the foundation of the first dental school in Baltimore, USA, the first dental magazine (*American Journal of Dental Science*), and the first dental society (American Society of Dental Science). In England, it was not until 1878 that the Dentist Act of that year gave the General Medical Council the power to examine and register suitably qualified dentists. However, it did not outlaw *un*qualified dentists, and you could still pull teeth out without any qualification at all. In 1880, with the founding of the British Dental Association, dentistry became a profession in Britain, and it was not until 1921 that unregistered dentists were outlawed. There are people alive today who may have had much of their early dental experience at the hands of a totally unqualified person.

In 1906 a school medical service was established which provided dental care for mothers and children of pre-school age, but, believe it or not, less than 2 per cent of the eligible population made use of this service. Most of the dentistry was carried out by dentists in private practice, although there were some dental hospitals in large cities. Dental disease was prevalent and, for the vast majority of the population, extraction was the only treatment for the relief of pain. Before the National Health Service, dentures were extremely expensive and many people had to go without, as old newsreel cuttings of the thirties and forties amply illustrate. (Indeed it is not so long since a full set of dentures was a prized twenty-first birthday present: today it might be a Mini!) Often the nervous middle-aged patient of today remembers bad experiences of the past – memories of austere waiting rooms and antiseptic smelling surgeries mingled with visions of bloody spittoons and treadle drills.

With dental disease so widespread, the dentist could easily become hardened to pain and suffering. His priorities were to remove as much infection from the mouth as possible, for, before the use of effective antibiotics, dental infections could be life-threatening. There *were* undoubtedly dentists who exhibited a caring and preventative approach, but the image created in the populace was one of fear.

With the inception of the National Health Service in 1948, dentistry became freely available to all, and there was a great demand for dental treatment which the profession could barely meet. Although the introduction of the high-speed drill in the fifties enabled the dentist to prepare tooth cavities rapidly for fillings, conservative dentistry consisted mainly of repair work because of this massive backlog. During this period, therefore, preventative dentistry was not practised effectively, and priority was given to ensuring patients were 'dentally fit'. The system of paying general dental practitioners has been called a treadmill by more than one commentator, because as more treatments were done by dentists working faster and more efficiently, the fee for that treatment would fall or at least would not be increased. So in order to earn the same money the dentist had to do *more* of those treatments. The effect of this was to encourage more direct treatment by making conservation more rewarding than extraction and to make more costly types of treatment less rewarding. But it also tended to encourage quantity rather than quality of treatment, and did not reward the dentist for teaching his patients about dental health and hygiene.

Since the 1970s, I feel that there has been an increasing emphasis on preventative dentistry and this has stemmed from undergraduate training and the employment by many general practitioners of dental hygienists and health educators. Dental officers now regularly visit schools to give advice and information to our children. Manufacturers of dental toothbrushes and pastes have also played an important part in delivering the message of prevention through various education campaigns and literature, often distributed free via the dental profession. It is encouraging to observe that there has been a reduction in tooth decay in the last ten years, and with this comes the hope that more resources can be channelled into a totally preventative system – the theme of this book.

It is curious to think that a service to treat disease was called a 'health service'. My hope for the future is that dentists can *truly* provide a 'health service', one that can educate, achieve, maintain and generally strive towards the health of the whole person.

CHAPTER TWO

The Anatomy of Teeth and Jaws

The formation of teeth and jaws is a top priority in nature's order of things and, astonishingly, the milk or baby teeth are already beginning to calcify or harden in the jaw of the embryo as early as ten weeks after conception, probably just when the pregnancy is being confirmed. Teeth are a priority organ because primitive man could not have survived without them – he would not have been able to eat – and even in times of severe hardship or malnutrition a baby will develop teeth. The bones of a starving child might show gross skeletal problems such as rickets, but the teeth – although they will probably be affected (by what dentally we call hypo-, or under-, calcification) – will still be present and will be in fairly adequate shape. The bones might be so affected that a child could not walk, but, in terms of nature's priorities, the teeth will form, thus would appear to be more important: it might not matter if a child can't walk, but it does if he can't chew.

Teeth and jaws, therefore, are a vital consideration right from the very start of life, and I shall cover this both here and in the next chapter. Firstly, I would like to describe the basic structures of teeth and jaws, and some factors that can affect their initial formation.

The Teeth

Mankind starts off with twenty milk or baby teeth, the deciduous teeth (and deciduous dentally means exactly the same as it does botanically: deciduous teeth are shed like the leaves from a tree). Thereafter we are the proud possessors of thirty-two permanent teeth. The variety of these teeth, at both stages of tooth development, shows clearly that man is an omnivore, that he does not have a specialization for eating either grass or meat. The incisors, or front teeth, are for cutting; the pointed canines are for tearing, revealing a meat-eating ancestry (like dogs and the big cats); and the molars at the back are the flat grinding teeth to cope with the chewing of tough raw meats, grasses and grains. All in all we have a pretty good jaw and set of teeth to cope with most types of food.

To define the teeth more clearly, it is easiest to use the approach of the dentist, in that dental language is a sort of scientific shorthand. This does not have to be learned by the lay reader, obviously, but it could help you understand a little more of what is going on the next time you go to the dentist!

The dentist divides the mouth up into quadrants, with each side possessing a matching number of teeth – five deciduous and eight permanent. When he specifies, say, the upper-left quadrant, he means left from the patient's point of view, not his own. In the UK, teeth are numbered from 1 to 8, using the very front tooth as 1 and the wisdom tooth as 8. Each quadrant of the mouth can then be described. Because the teeth are only duplicated on each side – there aren't any variations unless a tooth is missing – no quadrant is different from another basically, which immediately simplifies an understanding of the language of the mouth.

In further defining a tooth, six more points must be considered:

1   Is it a deciduous or permanent tooth?

2   Is it an incisor (1 or 2), a canine (3), a pre-molar (4 or 5), or a molar (6, 7 or 8)?

3   Is it maxillary (upper jaw) or mandibular (lower jaw)?

4   If it is an incisor, is it a central incisor (1) or a lateral incisor (2)?

5   If it is a pre-molar, is it a first (number 4, that nearest the front of the mouth) or second (5, the next one back)?

6   If it is a molar, is it a first (6), second (7) or third (8)?

Many of these particular questions depend, of course, on the age of the owner of the teeth: the first molars grow at around six years old; the second appear at about twelve; and the third, the wisdom teeth, appear usually in the late teens, early twenties.

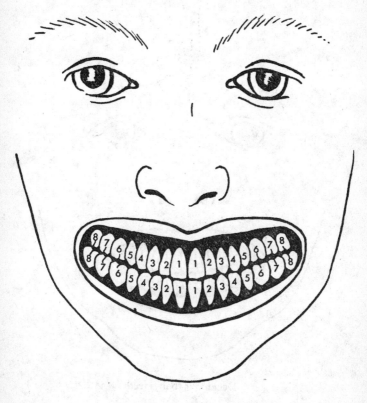

Permanent (adult) teeth

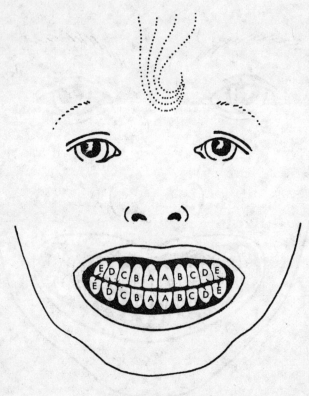

Deciduous (baby) teeth

In deciduous dentition, the terminology is slightly different. Although divided similarly into quadrants, the teeth are defined as A, B, C, D and E instead of 1–8. A baby has a central incisor (A), a lateral incisor (B), a canine (C), a first molar (D) and a second molar (E). Charts of the dates of eruption of both deciduous and permanent teeth are on pages 24 and 25.

Each tooth has a further five aspects, its surfaces, which are defined dentally: the top or biting surface is the occlusal; the side nearest the cheeks is the buccal; the side nearest the tongue is the lingual; the mesial is the surface nearest to the front of the mouth; and the distal is the surface furthest away from the front of the mouth. These again need not concern the lay reader too closely, but it will help when brushing your teeth to remember *five* surfaces ought to be cleaned!

The Structure of a Tooth

Each tooth is rooted into the gums and held firmly in place by the jawbone. In a healthy tooth there is no direct contact between root and bone: between them there is a layer of what we call periodontal fibres or ligaments which hold the teeth in the bone like little hammocks. You can test this yourself by moving one of your (hopefully) healthy teeth from side to side. Instead of the tooth being rigid, it will move a tiny bit, not because the bone is soft, but because of these fibres. The reason for this is that when we chew, we need a little 'give', otherwise chewing could be as unpleasant as riding on a bumpy road in a car with no suspension. In fact, the periodontal fibres are very much like a sophisticated suspension unit, and will become very much more relevant when we consider gum disease in Chapter Seven, because this is the layer often stripped away with disease, causing the tooth to be lost.

The root of the tooth is often much larger than the crown and, depending on what tooth it is, has one, two or three roots. Occasionally there are exceptions in the number and size. The root has canals flowing through it from the bone into the interior of the tooth. These contain blood vessels and nerve endings, and the little 'hole' where they join the bone proper is called the apical foramen. This hole is important both because of its channelling

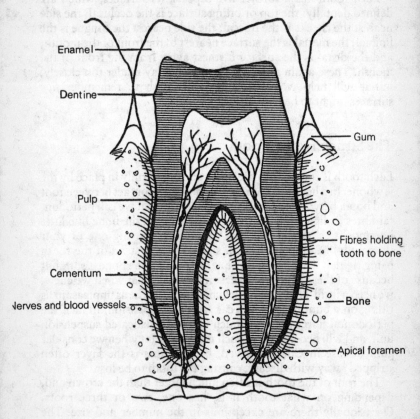

Structure of a tooth (molar)

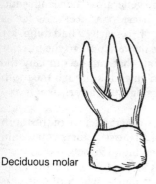

Deciduous molar

Permanent molar

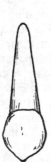

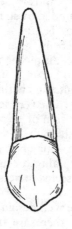

Deciduous canine

Permanent canine

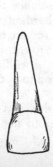

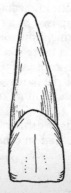

Deciduous incisor

Permanent incisor

functions, but also because its size can be constricted, especially with age – when of course you can get a generalized hardening and ageing of body tissue such as bone, arteries and teeth. As far as teeth are concerned, though, this is not necessarily a bad thing, for if there were to be a cutting off of the nerve supply to the interior pulp of the tooth, all the painful trials that can accompany the nerve endings of teeth are brought to an end (although the tooth will now suffer the tribulations of ageing, such as brittleness and colour changes etc.).

The pulp in the very interior is like the nerve centre of the tooth (in more ways than one). It consists of all the structures you would find within living tissue, such as nerves, blood vessels and connective tissue. The only tissue it lacks is muscle! One of the principal features of the pulp is its sensitivity to pain – which of course is why it is surrounded by so many protective layers. In the body in general, if tissue is hurt – a kick on the shins, say – it bruises, swells, and there is inflammation: the body is reacting, all its defences and repair mechanisms are rushing to the site. If pulp is damaged it also becomes inflamed. However, it cannot swell up because it is contained within a rigid structure, and the nerves are crushed and become very sensitive, and pain results. Pain, caused by the transmission of pressure on to nerve endings, occurs very quickly when the pulp is damaged, and because the outlet – the apical foramen – may be small this pressure can only be relieved slowly. This explains to a certain extent why pain in a tooth can be so severe, and seems to persist for such an interminable period of time.

But teeth are well designed in general, and to protect the pulp from damage, there are further layers – the dentine and the enamel. The one immediately around the pulp is dentine, which is basically composed of a substance similar to the outer layer, the enamel. Dentine, however, is less hard, of a much more organic composition, a more spaced-out structure in general. It has little tubules which contain mechanisms to register sensations such as pain, whereas the harder enamel is generally thought to be inert. Dentine is similar in its composition to bone, but is structurally different.

Dentine has a further security device, a property completely unique to it, and another pointer to the sheer efficiency and far-sightedness of the body and its mechanisms. Stone-age man's teeth often wore down very quickly because of the abrasive foods he ate: if the enamel wore through, first the dentine and then the pulp would be exposed. To help combat this – and it is still a sign of wear and tear, of ageing, in present-day teeth – the tooth lays down *more* dentine (called physiological or adventitious secondary dentine). This ensures that there is a longer time span before the attrition causes a painful pulp exposure. Hand in hand with age and this enlarging of the dentine layer goes the diminishing of the size of the pulp chamber.

The outer layer of the tooth – the most visible and therefore the one most people worry about – is the enamel. Enamel is the hardest substance in the body, and its major constituents are calcium and phosphate. It's similar to the material that makes bone as well, but the calcium for teeth is laid down in a crystalline form and this tends to give the hardness. As mentioned, enamel and dentine are similar in content, although formulated differently: there is 35 per cent calcium in enamel as opposed to 24 per cent in dentine; the organic content of enamel is 1.1 per cent as opposed to 21 per cent in dentine; there is 4 per cent water content in enamel, 10 per cent in dentine.

Enamel, although inert – lacking the sensation of pulp and dentine – is not as chemically stable as most people would believe. On the contrary, the surface of the enamel has a certain amount of permeability, meaning that there can be uptake into and loss from that surface, of both good things and bad. The older the tooth, the less permeable it becomes, whereas newly erupted or *young* teeth are more chemically active, permeable and therefore vulnerable. Should they be in an environment which produces a lot of acid – a mouth which, sadly, is all too common in the six to seven age group, when sweet-eating is often at its height – then the acids can attack the permeable enamel much more rapidly and start the process of tooth decay. However, fluoride is also clinically significant here. Just as the enamel can take up the acids, so it can take up 'topical' fluoride, that is any fluoride that may be present in the mouth, close to the tooth's surface. As topical fluoride *is* undoubtedly of benefit to teeth (other less beneficial aspects are discussed elsewhere), thus the permeability of the enamel can be used to advantage and can help prevent tooth decay: if, say, a new permanent molar is coated with fluoride shortly after eruption – at the age of six or seven – the uptake on the surface will probably be higher, therefore it will be more effective than it would be on that same tooth if it were left a few years to mature in the mouth.

The final layer in the tooth structure is the cement, which covers the root. The enamel layer normally joins the cement at what is called the cemento-enamel junction, and this is where the protective cement takes over. If this weren't there, the dentine would be exposed. However, in some 40 per cent of the population, the join of the cement does not coincide with the end of the enamel, and there is a little area where the three surfaces – enamel, dentine and cement – are side by side rather than overlapping. If gums are healthy and firm against the enamel on the side of the tooth, this may not cause too much trouble; if the 'seal' between the gum and tooth has been broken – because of incipient gum disease, say – then the dentine can be stimulated by acidic, sweet, hot or cold foods, or by the toothbrush filaments, and the result is what is commonly known as 'sensitive' teeth. This can also happen with age, as the gums recede; over-vigorous brushing can also wear away the cement and dentine as they are not so hard as the enamel.

Calcification

Given the complexity of the structural anatomy of the teeth, it is perhaps surprising that there are so *few* severe problems. But problems undoubtedly *do* occur, and the major ones involving the actual formation of teeth are those occurring during calcification or mineralization – during the *hardening* of the teeth. As this hardness is one of the properties unique to them, one of their most useful qualities, any weakening or abnormalities can be disastrous. Hypo-calcification (or *less* calcium than desirable) can result in teeth with nooks and crannies which can harbour bacteria, with surfaces which are less resistant to tooth decay – and of course, mechanically, they can break and chip more readily.

Teeth are basically composed of calcium phosphate, and the amount of this contained in enamel is greater than that found in the underlying dentine or indeed in bone. Comparatively speaking, enamel is harder than steel, being virtually the hardest forming natural substance. The actual composition of tooth is called a hydroxy apatite, and this has the chemical formula of $CA_{10}(PO_4)_6OH$. That sounds complicated, but its relevance is that, as with almost all chemical structures, the formula can be modified by the addition of other elements. There are other inorganic parts of the enamel and dentine and these, in element form, can be in terms of fluoride, lead, zinc, iron, chloride, sodium, magnesium, carbonate, strontium, copper, aluminium and potassium, to name but a few. Some, such as strontium, fluoride and zinc, can be relatively high in the tooth composition, while others are more in trace form. Lead, for instance, can show up in the teeth, and one way of testing for a dangerously high intake of lead, or for lead poisoning, might be to examine the shed deciduous teeth of children at risk.

From as early as the third month of pregnancy up to the age of five years, both deciduous and permanent teeth are calcifying (with the exception of wisdom teeth). During this period there are factors that may disturb the calcification, and I list some examples below. Diet is the classic one, and because I consider that so important, so central to my whole thesis, I discuss that separately thereafter.

1 Birth trauma can affect calcification. Birth is an extraordinarily busy time dentally and there are some forty-four teeth present, all in some stage of development – either the crowns or the roots. If the birth process is prolonged, or presents some difficulty or stress to the baby, the calcification is disturbed. Indeed, on most people if you look closely enough at their teeth, you can see what we call the neo-natal line, a fine line of marginal discoloration in the enamel, which charts the disturbance in the growing of the tooth when the actual birth took place. This line is horizontal to the axis of the tooth, and will affect all those teeth that are calcifying at the time of trauma. To illustrate the timing more clearly: at this stage, at birth, the first permanent molars – which don't erupt until about the age of six – are being calcified, and the line will show clearly on them. The effects can also show, particularly if the birth trauma was

Chronology of the deciduous teeth

Tooth	Initial calcification	Completion of crown	Eruption	Completion of roots
Upper first incisor	3–4 months in utero	4 months	7½ months	1½–2 years
Lower first incisor	4½ months in utero	4 months	6½ months	1½–2 years
Upper second incisor	4½ months in utero	5 months	8 months	1½–2 years
Lower second incisor	4½ months in utero	4½ months	7 months	1½–2 years
Upper canine	5 months in utero	9 months	16–20 months	2½–3 years
Lower canine	5 months in utero	9 months	16–20 months	2½–3 years
Upper first molar	5 months in utero	6 months	12–16 months	2–2½ years
Lower first molar	5 months in utero	6 months	12–16 months	2–2½ years
Upper second molar	6 months in utero	10–12 months	1¾–2½ years	3 years
Lower second molar	6 months in utero	10–12 months	1¾–2½ years	3 years

Adapted from chart based on the work of Logan and Krönfeld, reproduced in *Dental Morphology* by G. C. Van Beek (Wright Publishing Co., 1983)

Chronology of the permanent teeth

Tooth	Initial calcification	Completion of crown	Eruption	Completion of roots
Upper first incisor	3–4 months	4–5 years	7–8 years	10 years
Lower first incisor	3–4 months	4–5 years	6–7 years	9 years
Upper second incisor	10–12 months	4–5 years	8–9 years	11 years
Lower second incisor	3–4 months	4–5 years	7–8 years	10 years
Upper canine	4–5 months	6–7 years	11–12 years	13–15 years
Lower canine	4–5 months	6–7 years	9–10 years	12–14 years
Upper first premolar	1½–2 years	5–6 years	10–11 years	12–13 years
Lower first premolar	1¾–2 years	5–6 years	10–12 years	12–13 years
Upper second premolar	2–2½ years	6–7 years	10–12 years	12–14 years
Lower second premolar	2¼–2½ years	6–7 years	11–12 years	13–14 years
Upper first molar	Birth or slightly before	2½–3 years	6–7 years	9–10 years
Lower first molar	Birth or slightly before	2½–3 years	6–7 years	9–10 years
Upper second molar	2½–3 years	7–8 years	12–13 years	14–16 years
Lower second molar	2½–3 years	7–8 years	12–13 years	14–15 years
Upper third molar	7–9 years	12–16 years	17–21 years	18–25 years
Lower third molar	8–10 years	12–16 years	17–21 years	18–25 years

Adapted from chart based on the work of Logan and Krönfeld, reproduced in *Dental Morphology* by G. C. Van Beek (Wright Publishing Co., 1983) severe, on the front incisors – and they do not erupt until the age of seven or eight.

2 Antibiotics can affect calcification. The various forms of tetracycline – which are used for sore throats, chest infections and severe colds – can cause discoloration of the teeth. The tetracyclines are useful antibiotics because, apart from dentally, they don't have a lot of other side effects, but they ought not to be prescribed for women during pregnancy or lactation, nor for a child under the age of eight, by which time calcification is completely finished.

Calcium is laid down in the teeth in waves, like rings on a tree, with one layer landing on top of another. If a tetracycline is given during this formative time, it tends to target the calcium and thus give a horrendous banding of colour right through the layers. This can be very disfiguring, and sadly, because it's incorporated into the teeth rather than lying on the surface, it cannot be polished off. In very severe cases, when children are older, the dentist may need to crown the teeth or utilize the veneer techniques which we shall discuss later.

Different forms of tetracycline will produce different colours: aureomycin will produce a brown-grey (either or both); ledermycin, terramycin and actomycin will produce yellow stains. (Vibromycin is the only one which doesn't have this discolouring effect.) On the eruption of the tooth and its exposure to ultra-violet light – sunlight – the colour change appears. The teeth can also be affected by varying degrees of hypo-calcification so, with less calcium in the tooth than needed, the tooth will be structurally weaker.

3 Another 'colour-change merchant' affecting calcification is fluoride. I discuss fluoride in much greater detail later on, in Chapter Six, in relation to tooth decay, but its deleterious effect on tooth formation isn't often admitted by those who lobby for the fluoridation of water supplies. Fluoride is a mineral known to deprive the body of calcium, and if ingested excessively during the tooth calcification process, not surprisingly it interferes to a greater or lesser extent with it.

Fluorosis (the abnormalities caused to the teeth by too much fluoride ingested during this period) is becoming increasingly common in our society. As anything above two parts per million – fluoride to water – is considered potentially hazard-ous, and with fluoride in drinking water, in toothpastes, in drops, tablets and topical treatments (it's even contained in tea), many children at the vulnerable stage can be getting far too much.

In mild overdosage there is a lustreless opaque appearance to the enamel – which should gleam and shine – and it lies either in patches or over the whole tooth. In more severe cases the teeth can be stained yellow and brown, with mottled enamel creating pits in the surface which can be havens for the tooth decay bacteria. In extreme cases of fluorosis, you can actually get a complete shape change of the tooth as well, with extensive hypoplasia (under-calcification). So, although in theory the fluoride may render the tooth more resistant to tooth decay, in reality fluoride can be one of the most serious disfiguring elements for teeth.

4 If the mother contracts syphilis, she can pass it on to her baby in the womb, and it is the permanent teeth that are more usually affected: deficient or missing enamel, poorly formed dentine, and the incisors are often shaped rather like crescents. How-ever, due to the use of antibiotics and a greater awareness of the dangers of the disease, dentists do not often see patients display-ing these signs nowadays.

5 There is a genetic association with abnormal calcification, and this is literally when a family's genes produce bad forma-tion of the tooth structure. Just as a mother's 'gappy' teeth might reproduce genetically in her children, so a parent's tendency to weak teeth or thin enamel can be reproduced as well. In *amelo genesis imperfecta*, the enamel is affected; in *dentino genesis imperfecta*, it's the dentine that is affected. This latter can almost be worse than damaged enamel: as the underlying structure of the tooth is weak, the tooth can collapse in upon itself once it starts to be used. These are rare con-ditions.

6 Childhood illnesses such as measles, chickenpox and scarlet fever – all of which are likely to produce fevers or general disruption in the whole body – will also cause abnormalities if they occur during the years of calcification. Sadly, of course, these years – from birth to about four or five – are the ones in

which children most commonly fall prey to a host of ailments. With so many suffering to a greater or lesser degree from colds, snuffles, flu, raised temperatures etc., it's not surprising therefore, when you look carefully at the teeth of both older children and adults – especially the incisors which are easier to examine – that there are so many visible flaws in the enamel: little white or coloured marks and changes in the opacity, giving rise to a colour which is not consistent. If the illness was long and severe, it can mean that the teeth that are calcifying at that time can be virtually ruined, in the sense that the calcium is laid down badly and haphazardly, sometimes not laid down at all.

7   The final thing that can commonly affect calcification is local infection or trauma. This occurs at a later stage – in the first two years, say – and a classic instance is when a child falls over and bashes his front baby teeth, pushing them up in the jaw. If they rise far enough, this can physically affect the germ of the second tooth above, and if this is not fully calcified at the time, it will be damaged. Similarly, if a child gets early tooth decay, with a dental abscess, say, on a baby tooth, the development of the permanent tooth beneath can be affected as well.

NUTRITION AND CALCIFICATION

To put it simply, correct nutrition is the very foundation of health for the whole body, let alone the teeth. A good maternal diet during pregnancy and lactation, and for the child, especially during that approximate four-year calcification period, is an investment for the whole future of the child and of his teeth. At no other time does growth take place quite so quickly as in the womb and in the first years of life, and so it is of paramount importance that the body cells get the maximum support and help from food, which is, of course, what is required to *make* them grow.

A good diet will ensure that jaws and other bones achieve their maximum potential, that teeth are formed well, and that calcification is as complete as possible. Hand in hand with this will obviously go general health, which will lessen the vulnerability to infections of all kinds for both mother and child, thus immediately getting rid of many of the causes of calcification abnormalities mentioned above. General health and good formation of teeth will also lessen the susceptibility to tooth decay because well formed teeth and jaws and well calcified teeth are more resistant to attack.

Calcium phosphate is the major constituent of both tooth and bone – about 99 per cent of the calcium in our bodies is in bones and teeth (the rest is for proper contraction of the muscles) – and fortunately calcium is very commonly found in food (even modern food). Unless a diet is very peculiar or unbalanced, it's not often that there is a serious deprivation, but we occasionally find effects on teeth which can be the direct result of insufficient calcium in the diet. Those most at risk are growing children and pregnant or lactating mothers. If the mother's diet is low in calcium, she may lose calcium from her bones, not from her teeth. There may be a greater likelihood of gum disease, but this is brought about by hormonal changes, rather than by calcium loss as is commonly believed. The baby will not suffer as *soon* as the mother – his demands have priority – but in extreme deprivation of calcium, poor skull and bone development as well as poor teeth can be a result.

Calcium is contained in such diverse things as milk and other dairy products (cheese and yoghurt particularly) and canned sardines! Milk, of course, is what is normally recommended for pregnant mothers in order that they may build up their calcium reserves. I believe, though, along with other nutritional practitioners, that the calcium of doorstep milk is often not in the best form for easy digestion, and the milk itself contains additives, so it may not be the best source. Green leafy vegetables, other vegetables such as carrots, and whole grains also contain calcium, and they should provide adequate supplies.

The average daily uptake of calcium is 0.8 g, while pregnant and lactating women normally need between 1.5–2 g. The overall amount of calcium in a new-born baby is 25 g; from birth to about 10 months, it goes up to 43 g; by the end of the first year there's a massive leap to 83 g – illustrating very dramatically that during periods of rapid growth (pregnancy and that first year), there is a very much larger requirement for calcium. Fortunately, those extra needs are met by the body which can extract greater amounts of the mineral from food eaten: thus the amount of absorption from the stomach and the amount that is actually utilized by the body can be regulated in such times of need. In fact all animals — including children — absorb greater proportions of calcium when growing, and even adults apparently vary their calcium uptake seasonally — an interesting thought, which might be a throwback to when diet might change seasonally, when there might not be enough food through the winter — or perhaps something to do with breeding cycles? Indeed, during the latter months of human pregnancy, of the extra amounts of calcium that are absorbed, only half goes into the baby: the other half goes into the bones of the mother. Basically we presume that this is in order that she will have a reserve for lactation, for bones are very active in terms of minerals flowing to and fro from them. It's actually hormonal changes that will alter the uptake of calcium, so again it's a controlled mechanism.

The main problem with calcium is absorption, and only part of that which we eat is absorbed. It all depends yet again on good diet in general, and certain vitamins in particular. A wrong diet can lead to malabsorption; so even though a mother, say, might be having the right quantity of calcium in her diet, because of other dietary factors leading to a wrong combination in her body, that calcium will be poorly absorbed.

Vitamin D is essential for the mechanism controlling absorption of calcium (as well as for the metabolism). It occurs in relatively few foods — in fish, margarine, eggs, dairy foods and liver only — and cod-liver oil, the bane of many a child's life, is the major source. Fortunately our skin manufactures D when exposed to sunlight, and if the summer months supply us with a certain proportion of our D requirements, diet needs to be relied upon for the rest of the year. Asians and West Indians living in Britain, whose dark skins were designed to protect them from a stronger sun, are not able to manufacture D in the weaker northern sun, so they may need D supplements. (Older people, too, suffer from lack of D: they wrap themselves up, stay indoors to keep warm, and don't get enough sunshine as a result.)

A deficiency of D in general, because it is so vital in the absorption and use of calcium, can cause bones to become brittle, and teeth to be ultimately lost. D is the vitamin most closely associated with rickets and osteomalacia, which means that when a child stands, the leg bones can bend and cause permanent deformity. Dentally, with a serious D deficiency, teeth can be hypoplastic – badly formed – but there is no conclusive evidence of this. Research has also suggested that D can help *prevent* tooth decay: it may be that D present in the saliva (for common or garden spit is very much more important than might be thought, see Chapter Four) enhances the oral environment, and lessens the chances of decay developing.

Supplementary vitamin drops – of A, C and D – are recommended in Britain for babies from five weeks, and can continue up to seven years. A full dose is five drops daily, although the British err on the side of safety: the Americans give very much more. Vitamin D overdoses can damage, however, and can even lead to death. Dentally they can cause ankylosis, where the bone cements around the tooth: that means that if the tooth had to be removed, part of the bone of the jaw would have to be removed as well. Excess D is also believed to cause pulp stones – little calcium stones which form in the pulp, and which can constrict the nerves and blood vessels flowing into the tooth.

Vitamins A and C as well as other minerals such as magnesium and zinc and many trace elements are also vital to the calcification process – as they are indeed to health generally. But it must be emphasized, though, that it is all a matter of balance, of a correct combination, and the only way in which this can be truly ensured is through a correct and sensible diet.

A number of things can *interfere* in a dietary sense with the absorption of calcium, and thus with the calcification process. Rickets and osteomalacia – direct results of defects of calcium metabolism in the tissues – are found in Britain in some children from the Indian sub-continent. Another contributory factor, however, is thought to be their chapatis, a basic bread made from a hard wholewheat flour, and a consistent part of their diet. The flour is high in phitates, which slow up the absorption of calcium and can actually leach calcium from the body, along with other minerals like magnesium. Research has shown that when chapatis were removed from these people's diets for a period of time as short as seven weeks, there was a marked *rise* in the calcium levels in their bodies. This is interesting in showing how a diet based on one food in large proportions can have a deleterious effect on the body, but even more so when one considers recent fads like high-fibre diets. Dietary fibre is undeniably essential for health, but an over-emphasis on the basics of such a diet – brown rice, brown bread, and especially bran, all of which are high in phitates – can have a very marked effect on the body. Although the body, being an adaptable organ, *can* become accustomed to a high-phitate diet, there is quite a large and rapid drain of calcium at first. And the main significance is that dangers could lie in over-enthusiastic parents putting their growing children on such a diet: calcium loss at such a time would be hazardous, and immature digestive systems would not be able to cope anyway.

Another factor affecting calcium absorption is the oxalic acid contained in such foods as spinach and rhubarb. Despite Popeye, and the powers given him by spinach, both foods should be avoided or at least limited in the diets of growing children and expectant mothers.

Finally, as regards diet and calcification, it does appear that a high-protein diet can *help* the absorption of calcium, as can the sugar or lactose in breast milk. I'm not necessarily recommending a high protein consumption, but it has some value in this area, although it also aids the excretion of calcium. But I am unreservedly recommending breast-feeding, as mother's milk is by far the best food any baby can have, not least because it will help in the calcification process.

The Jaw

From the dental point of view the jaw is the foundation stone, so to speak, of the whole dental configuration, and without its efficient working movements – opening, closing and chewing – many would not be able to survive. If food is not chewed properly, it affects the whole digestive system. It has been shown that when food is placed directly into the stomach, the experimental animal will become ill; if the same food is then chewed thoroughly in the mouth, taken out and placed in the stomach, the animal recovers its health.

Interestingly, just as teeth have priority over bone – and even in severe nutritional crises, do not easily yield their minerals (thus, accordingly, their hardness) – so nature has built safeguards into the jaw. Although we tend to think of babies as being quite helpless – unlike most other animal babies – they do still have certain birth reflexes. The Moro reflex is one: this occurs when a baby, thinking he is about to be dropped, will jerkily splay his limbs and grab with his hands, an echo, it is thought, of when the baby clung to his mother's fur; the fisting of the baby's hands around a finger is another. Dentally, though, the jaw will reflexively open and close without any control from the upper brain: a baby does not have to be 'taught' to suck or chew, the instinct is already there. In fact, even if all the nerves that control the jaw were cut – in an accident, say, with the victim a virtual 'living vegetable' – the body would react instinctively to the stimulation of something between the lips and teeth, and would open, close and chew (albeit only after a fashion). Nourishment of the body has priority yet again.

The jaw begins to form in the foetus even earlier than do the teeth: from about the fourth week after conception, certainly before any knowledge of pregnancy, the tissue which will become the arches of the jaw and palates is growing. The growth and formation of the jaw after a baby is born, and throughout the child's whole growing period, are modelled by specialized cells known as osteoblasts and osteoclasts: the former make the bone grow, *deposit* bone, and the latter dissolve bone. It is these cells, too, which are stimulated to make the teeth move through the jaw, both in the transition from deciduous to permanent teeth, and in the period when orthodontic treatments – braces and other dental appliances – may have to play a part. This constant activity and mobility means that the alveolar bones in the jaw, the ones that actually hold the teeth in place, are much more flexible than an adult's, and remain so throughout the whole growing period. This flexibility comes in handy when children go through their falling over and bumping faces period – they don't do nearly as much damage as an adult might, undergoing the same trauma – and may be nature's way of compensating for those years of instability and accidents. But this flexibility also accounts for many basic shaping mechanisms, which we call applied external pressure.

The most fundamental of these mechanisms is the one which actually forms the nice arcs of the upper and lower jaws and teeth. This is due to the lips and tongue which act like physical barriers to contain the teeth: the tongue pushes the teeth outwards towards the lip, and the lips and cheeks push the teeth inwards towards the tongue. If a growing child – and it is rare – had only part of a tongue, then the teeth and jaw bone on that side would tend to veer in towards the area that had no tissue to push them out again (a malformation of this basic shaping mechanism can occur with a thumbsucker who will pull the top arch out and push the bottom one in). Even a baby who lies on one side all the time can depress that side of the face and jaw so that he may look a little lopsided for a while – but this will soon be outgrown. Another basic shaping factor is feeding from the breast: proper sucking at the breast – the system designed by nature – will promote the best shape and development of the jaw and facial bone structure, and of the facial musculature in general.

But one of the major factors controlling jaw and teeth is still thought to be genetic. The size of the jaw, the shape, whether the teeth are big or small, whether they are well spaced within the jaw, can all be inherited from parents. A father's gap between his front teeth can be reproduced in his children; as can a mother's square or pointed chin and jaw. The 'class' of jaw can be inherited too. This is of significance dentally in orthodontics, and refers to the 'bite' of the teeth, how the upper and lower teeth come together in the jaw: class 1 is where the teeth meet virtually edge to edge; class 2 is where the top teeth protrude beyond the bottom teeth, and class 3 is where the bottom teeth stick out beyond the top teeth. Class 1 is generally considered to be the ideal, but in fact it's rare in western civilization to have a normal 'occlusion', to use the dental term. It's interesting, too, that we make assumptions about people based on class of jaw; an exaggerated class 2 and a small chin are almost invariably associated with 'chinless wonders' or 'upper-class twits'; a severe class 3 – a jutting-out lower jaw – is probably the worst malocclusion, and is the caricature 'hard case', suggesting aggression and dimness. Jaw class can also run in families. One of the most famous is that of the Habsburgs, the most prominent European imperial dynasty from the fifteenth to the twentieth centuries: from portraits, we can clearly see the classic class 3 or over-lantern jaw. But class of jaw can also be a racial characteristic: many Chinese or Japanese have class 2 bites; a slight class 3 is quite commonly seen in Scots!

It is when genetic or racial types are mixed that problems can occur dentally: a father with large jaw and teeth plus mother with small jaw and small teeth can produce a child with small jaw and large teeth. With large teeth crammed together in a jaw too small to properly accommodate them, the child will be prey to all the problems that are associated with crowding – difficulty in cleaning properly between tight teeth, thus a vulnerability to bacterial invasion followed by tooth decay and gum disease. This genetic aspect of jaw shape and its relationship with tooth crowding and decay was what was taught to me as an undergraduate at dental school; this was considered to be virtually the *only* cause of tooth crowding and thus a major contributory factor to tooth decay. Although much was taught on the relationship between tooth decay and diet, there was little consideration of the relationship between diet and crowded jaws. That this is still so, some fifty years after the findings of Dr Weston Price, an American dentist, seems unbelievable to me. *Nutrition and Physical Degeneration* was published in the thirties, and has become a bible, the foundation stone of their beliefs, for many nutritionists the world over. Dr Price investigated about fourteen primitive peoples worldwide – peoples who were pure bred, who had little contact with the outside world, and who were living on traditional, tribal, unprocessed and unrefined foods. They included Australian Aborigines, Alaskans, Polynesians, Eskimos, people living in remote Swiss valleys and in the high mountains of Peru, and, although there was an enormous diversity of races, tribal customs and native foods, Dr Price observed everywhere perfect teeth and good jaw and skeletal structures. He found a great change in these peoples, however, after they came in contact with civilization and with 'civilized' foods – white sugar and flour etc. Within one generation only – and the effects exhibited themselves with a *horrifying* rapidity – the people were suffering quite visibly from tooth decay and from a narrowing of jaws and dental arches. His book is filled with before and after photographs which illustrate dramatically – and with no possible doubt – how damaging modern refined foods can be, and how inextricably linked are nutrition and dental health.

The first important fact about Dr Price's work is its unique timeliness. Historically speaking, the decade in which he made and reported his findings was undoubtedly the last in which anyone had an opportunity to study such isolated communities. For one cannot now find any part of the world in which the peoples and their diets have not been basically altered to a greater or lesser extent by the 'advances' of civilization – by refined foods, by fertilizers, by drugs and chemicals, by pollution. Even in the thirties he encountered these peoples on the cusp, so to speak, being able to record their health verbally and photographically, both dentally and generally, before and after the introduction of modern ideas and foods – at the intervention of civilization.

The second factor that I consider vital is that he recorded so many different races. He did not look at just one or two peoples who perhaps were physiologically weaker or stronger, or who geographically were able to enjoy a better or worse diet (Eskimos ate meat almost exclusively; some had a mixed diet; some were virtually vegetarian): he looked at a huge variety in every sense, and everywhere he noted a superlative health which then degenerated in an astonishingly short time. He was looking at generation upon generation of pure-bred people, peoples not affected by the cross-breeding of racial types found in the northern hemisphere generally. In all cases he recorded good dental arches, good facial formations, broad nasal arches and wide jaws; yet within ten to fifteen years, these had all changed, and many of the younger people looked as if they belonged to a different tribe.

With the introduction of modern food – the sugars particularly – the first deterioration was that of tooth decay. The second most noticeable factor was that the developing children then suffered from malocclusions or bad growth of the jaws, with teeth crowded as a result. This occurred almost immediately, not just in the womb but exhibiting itself also in three- and four-year-olds who, by the time they were twelve, were showing crowding, decay and jaw degeneration that had never before been seen in family or group. Many also exhibited a rapid deterioration in their resistance to disease. In this pre-antibiotic era, tuberculosis still existed but, because of a good natural resistance in individuals, it was not common: among many of those, however, who showed most degeneration in teeth and jaws, it became a severe problem. Dr Price also recorded behavioural changes.

Some of his conclusions can, with justification, be criticized, but I believe this is principally due to the decade in which he was working: his grasp of the interaction of vitamins and minerals was good, for instance, but in the late thirties he lacked knowledge of the detailed research that has gone on since. In general, however, he shows in an extraordinarily graphic way the profound effect that diet can have on health, and raises the horrifying question of, if undeniably strong genetic bases can be *so visibly* affected, and so rapidly, by diet, what about the changes that cannot be so easily registered? What might be happening internally?

CHAPTER THREE

The Secret of Healthy Teeth for our Children

How can we guarantee that our children have good teeth? And where do we start? If dentistry becomes primarily preventative – as I hope most sincerely it does – then good advice must be given from the very beginning, and the utmost care must be taken by the parents right from that caricature initial twinkle in the father's eye onwards. It is the only way in which we can ensure the health of future generations.

Pre-Conceptual Care

It seems to me one of life's greatest ironies that, although commercial livestock and show animal breeders – even *hamster* breeders! – believe in a special programme and diets before breeding to ensure normal and healthy young, future human parents do not seem to give much thought to the health of their own bodies in relation to that of their potential offspring. Only in primitive societies, many of which were studied by Dr Weston Price, do we find any real evidence of this pre-conceptual concern. He recorded that in many different races, when a couple reached an age where they were thinking of having children, they were often put on special diets, given the best meats and the best and freshest foods in general. Thus they could be both more fertile, and their sperm and ova would have the best nutrition possible in order, hopefully, to produce the strongest offspring. They believed – and in the light of present-day knowledge, how can we deny it? – that they could help improve the quality of the species and produce a better and healthier next generation. With such apparent genetic sophistication, it is even more grossly ironic that these peoples should have fallen victim to the 'evils' of western civilization as described in the previous chapter.

It really goes without saying that the healthier the parents have been throughout their lives, and the healthier they are in the months prior to conception, then the healthier the baby. Many nutritionists nowadays believe that the bodies of both father and mother should be primed for at least two years prior to conception, and at the forefront of research and practice in Britain is Foresight, the Association for the Promotion of Pre-Conceptual Care. To a large extent the thinking behind Foresight has been inspired by the researches of Weston Price in the thirties, but the conclusions have been put very strongly and ably into practice on a much more scientific basis. Instead of relying totally upon the principles of good diet – although these are central to their aims and to the advice given by them – they also undertake many tests on prospective parents who attend their clinics.

A full medical history is taken and relevant factors are noted, like allergies, illnesses, forms of contraception used, and whether the mother has had German measles. They take all the usual tests – blood, urine, faeces, thyroid function, semen, and smear – and perform a hair analysis (the latter, important for fathers as well, can give a good insight into mineral and metal levels and deficiencies, during the three or so months of the hair growth). They even monitor other environmental factors such as drinking water, checking water at both home and work if hair samples have shown any metal contamination in excess of the World Health Organization limit. Foresight also recommend pre-conceptual supplements for both parents, marketing three different varieties which contain a very wide range of vitamins and minerals, and publish helpful leaflets. By this general health screening, of course, any factors which could hamper fertility or which could cause defects in a future baby can be brought to light, examined, referred on to general medical practitioners or specialists, and remedied if possible before conception.

A planned pregnancy is the most sensible of all, for before a mother even realizes she has missed her first period, she may have encountered many substances – whether environmental or dietary – which might be harmful to the growing child. For it must never be forgotten that, during that first six to eight weeks after conception, all the organs of the body, limbs, face, jaw and teeth begin their separate development. This pre-conceptual care is, I think, absolutely vital, and in this area holistic dentists could play a significant part. If newly-married couples came, say, to the surgery to be checked, the dentist could ask them if they were thinking of starting a family. If the answer were affirmative, he could offer them advice, give them some pointers to health, literature on nutrition, refer them on to organizations like Foresight. He might even ultimately be enabled to do some of the tests himself. The dentist, seeing people at regular intervals, is in an extremely strong position to monitor general health, and to step in with significant advice at such appropriate times.

POINTERS TO PRE-CONCEPTUAL HEALTH

1 If a prospective mother has not had German measles, she should be immunized against the disease at least three months before conception. This avoids the risks of babies being born with hearing and other defects.

2 If a prospective mother is on the contraceptive pill, she should change to an alternative method of contraception at least four to six months before planning to conceive in order to reduce risk of miscarriage and defects (the pill also reduces the mother's levels of Vitamin C and iron). Those using the copper coil should change contraceptive method at about the same time.

3 If drugs are taken in connection with diseases such as diabetes, eczema, asthma, migraine or epilepsy, then the parents, especially the mother, should seek a doctor's advice at least three months before conception. As drug-taking should be completely avoided during pregnancy, advance consideration should be given to alternatives. Foresight also advise in this area.

4 If either parent smokes, particularly the mother, they should try to stop before conception. The physical manifestations of nicotine withdrawal – as well as the psychological ones – can be very distressing, so it's more sensible to do this now. It should

most particularly be avoided during pregnancy, but as it so profoundly affects all the cells and tissue of the body, it can only do good to cut it out at this stage.

5 Follow a sensible wholefood diet, avoiding as much as possible any excesses such as alcohol. Fresh fruit and vegetables, preferably raw, should be eaten at least once daily – they are rich in vitamins and minerals. The less fatty protein sources such as liver, poultry, and fish should be eaten two or three times a week. Eat plenty of whole grains, nuts and pulses, and for snacks, eat dried fruits as opposed to sweets or cakes. Remember to try to boost the calcium reserves even at this stage. Avoid fat as much as possible, either visible as on meat, or that which is hidden in butter, cheese, whole milks etc. Avoid salt as much as possible, and sugar at all costs!

6 Mothers should take as much exercise as they can in the months prior to pregnancy: exercise of any kind tones up the body in general and benefits the heart and lungs in particular. Gentle floor or yoga exercises are particularly helpful for relaxing mind and body. Remember that anything now is valuable, but too much exercise during the actual pregnancy can sometimes be harmful. Fresh air is important too, for oxygen is as much a nutrient of the body as is good food.

Pre-Natal Care

Once conception has taken place, the onus is on the mother to make her body the most ideal environment in which her baby can grow and flourish to his fullest potential. More than at any other time, her diet is absolutely crucial, for what she ingests is what will pass through her body to her baby; his teeth and bone structure, general mental and physical health, freedom from allergies and intellectual potential, although to an extent governed by heredity, are in the main dependent upon maternal diet during his nine months spent in the womb. The womb environment can also be damaged or modified, however, by factors other than diet, and the mother has to constantly maintain her scrupulous guardianship of her growing baby, censoring all the substances, environmental and other hazards that I list below.

Once again, the dentist could be at the forefront of medical care at this stage. A dentist's knowledge of a patient's pregnancy is vital anyway, in a number of ways: as dental work is free in Britain during pregnancy and for a year afterwards, many mothers take advantage of that fact and attend more regularly; as pregnancy does undoubtedly cause some mothers distinct dental problems, they will probably *need* to consult the dentist; and as X-rays are thought to be hazardous to the growing baby, the dentist will have to be informed before undertaking any treatment involving X-rays etc. These are but a few of the factors directly related to dentistry, but a good holistic dentist could also be giving dietary advice, and keeping an eye on how his patient and patient-to-be are progressing. Health care in general at this time is, of course, very good, with doctors, ante-natal clinics, health visitors etc. monitoring and contributing health and dietary advice. But few even now are specialists in nutrition as such – although organizations like Foresight are available – and this is undoubtedly where a nutritionally trained dentist could play a part. Indeed there's no reason why the same advice should not come from all sources – the more the merrier in fact. It's indubitably true of life, but particularly true when you're a first-time mother, that the greater the number of professional people who agree on a subject relating to you – in this case, a good diet – the more likely you are to follow that advice, and the more assured you will be that you are doing the right thing.

The dentist could be utilized much more as yet another health 'screen', so to speak. If he has a good relationship with his patient, often a relaxed conversation between them can clear up many a point thought to be too trivial to bother a doctor with. If he keeps a full medical history of his patient – and I believe every dentist should – then he can reassure on and back up normal medical advice on such things as high blood pressure, diabetes etc. He could be the one to spot an anaemia or vitamin deficiency in a pregnant patient, and he would also spot weight abnormalities. He could look out for some of the danger signs such as alcoholism, smoking or drug-taking, and he can give advice on such maternal vagaries as pica, the craving for eating inedible substances such as coal! With so many teenaged pregnancies these days, he could advise here strongly on diet, for the teenage proclivity for hamburgers and fizzy drinks could be very detrimental to health of mother *and* baby. Although pregnancy is a prime time for health care in this country, the dentist ought to be enabled to play a much more positive and all-round role.

A HEALTHY DIET DURING PREGNANCY

That good maternal diet is the most fundamental factor of a healthy baby, both bodily and dentally, is undisputed on every level of medical practice. In fact there is a definite relationship between poor nutrition and the poor physical growth of the foetus, especially in the development of the lower brain section which is associated with coordination and general physical ability. The teeth, as already outlined, take priority over bone when there are dietary deficiencies. They *will* be formed – present-day children in Ethiopia, for instance, who are suffering from the severest malnutrition, are born with workable teeth – but they may not be in as good condition as they might be.

The mother's own long-term health is dependent on her diet at this time too, and there is no reason why she should lose her teeth and her figure and end up with unsightly varicose veins, stretch marks and wrinkles of fatigue. There is no need either, despite the old belief, to 'eat for two'; that would lead to an unnecessary weight gain that will be difficult to shed afterwards. A certain gain is, of course, necessary to allow for the growth of the baby, for the fat deposits to be used for breast feeding, for the placenta and amniotic fluid etc. The average total gain required is about 18 lb (8 kg), and more than 20–24 lb (9–12 kg) would indicate undesirable excess fat or fluid retention. The need during pregnancy is for increased nutrients, not increased calories – even in mid term a mother only needs about an extra 300 calories a day – and extra bulk like buns can only have a detrimental effect on the mother's teeth, and won't do the baby any good, or the mother's figure after birth.

Although I go on below to specify many vitamins and minerals that are desirable for bodily and dental health at this time, it must be emphasized that it is the overall *balance* of the diet that is important. If the right foods are eaten, and carefully considered in relationship with each other, all the necessities will be ingested in the most natural way, thus obviating the need for supplementation. Many pregnant mothers used to be given supplements of iron, for instance. Iron is undoubtedly needed during pregnancy, as the baby has to take enough from his mother to see him through the months in the womb and the first few months of life, and too little iron in the maternal diet could thus lead to maternal anaemia. But at the same time, too much iron – when there is tablet supplementation, say – could interfere with the absorption and use of other minerals and trace elements such as magnesium and zinc, which are equally as important in their way. Similarly, although pregnancy can be a time when constipation is a problem, by over-enthusiastic consumption of bran or other high-fibre foods, the Vitamin D, and thus calcium, absorption could be diminished. *Balance* must be the key word, and if it sounds as if you should have a chemistry degree before giving birth, don't worry: follow a few simple rules, and rely on a good healthy diet which should do it all for you!

Proteins. These are required for growth and repair of all the organs of the body, and most people in the northern hemisphere probably get more than enough. The approximate daily protein requirement of an expectant mother is about 2 oz (50 g), and that is contained in a couple of slices of good wholemeal bread or a cup of milk: an 8 oz (225 g) steak is clearly over-indulgence. Too much meat during pregnancy anyway can mean too large a phosphorus intake which can lead to leg cramps. Complete proteins, which supply a complete range of amino acids (the constituents of protein), are supplied by milk (human, animal and dried), meat, poultry, fish, eggs, cheese and yoghurt, and soya beans (the only food of non-animal origin that is a complete protein). Incomplete proteins supplying a limited range of amino acids, are usually cheaper and are contained in whole grains and all products made from them such as pasta and bread, in dried beans, peas and lentils etc., and in nuts and seeds.

Holistically, I believe that many sources of complete protein should be questioned, for it's the *quality* of the food that counts: meats nowadays contain additives, and the meat-producing animals are given growth hormones; milk and cheese also contain additives; eggs and poultry should be free-range, and fish is perhaps the only complete protein that is as yet free of tampering (although pollution could be taking its toll, as it has already in the Mediterranean). Vegetables, however, if grown organically and are unsprayed, will supply good protein, and a variety of the incomplete proteins will see most expectant mothers – especially vegetarians who need to be particularly careful to have sufficient protein – happily through pregnancy.

Fats. Everyone should be careful about fat consumption, but a *moderate* amount is needed during periods of growth. Research suggests that essential fatty acids are needed in tooth formation – those provided by fish oils and unheated sunflower and safflower oils etc. – but the major role of fats and oils in diet, and particularly at this stage, is that they are responsible for the absorption of the fat-soluble vitamins A, D, E and K.

Vitamins. The necessity for Vitamin D has already been discussed. The other vitamins given as drops to babies are A and C, and they are important dentally during pregnancy. A is important both for the formation of the tooth enamel and for the connective tissue or collagen. An A deficiency can affect the osteoblasts, the cells that deposit or make bone, thus teeth, jaws and other bones are affected. A is contained in animal and fish livers (cod liver oil is the major source) and dairy foods in one form, and in a second form, beta-carotene, in green, yellow and orange vegetables and fruit (carrots, spinach and dried apricots in particular). A is poisonous, like D, in too large doses.

Vitamin C cannot be manufactured in the human body, although of course we can ingest it. Animals can manufacture it, however, and Dr Weston Price, when studying peoples who lived in the snowy wastes of the north, found that, in the absence of C in fruit or vegetable form, they had learned to eat certain glands of the animals they killed – the adrenals – which contained the vitamin. C is involved in tooth formation and is vital in the building of tissue structures such as collagen. It is very strongly linked with iron, as mentioned, and a lack of C at this time can interfere with the action of the osteoblasts. The classic – historic even – dental disturbance associated with a deficiency of C is scurvy. This disease can develop astonishingly quickly and it has been shown that, on the sea voyages plagued by the disease –

before the advent of the curative lemon – the gums of sailors became swollen and red after 30 weeks only. Even babies can develop a form of scurvy, which basically exhibits itself as bleeding gums, and there can also be gross swelling and ulceration. Holistic dentists use Vitamin C in large doses to slow down the progress of gum disease, and C also aids quick recovery from injury and operations etc. It is thus very strongly linked with the gums and the tissues that hold the teeth in the jaw.

C is found in fresh fruit and vegetables, and is water soluble, so cooking should be avoided whenever possible. But, although it is undeniably important, it should not be taken in mega doses during pregnancy. The baby could actually suffer after birth from C 'withdrawal', believe it or not. With such a high level of the vitamin circulating while he was in the womb, he could develop a low C level and scurvy symptoms in the months *after* birth.

The B vitamin group – B_1 (thiamin), B_2 (riboflavin), nicotinic acid (niacin in the US), pantothenic acid, B_6 (pyridoxine), B_{12} (cyanocobalamine), and folic acid – are all important in general during pregnancy, major sources being yeast extract, wheatgerm and liver. With deficiencies of many of these, the mouth and tongue can be affected. In pregnancy, however, a deficiency of B_6 and B_{12} can cause anaemia, but a proper intake of B_6 can reduce nausea, fatigue, dizziness and leg cramps. B_{12} does not occur in plants in large amounts, and thus vegetarian mothers should take supplements. Folic acid is perhaps the most important, though, for a deficiency has been shown to be a major causative factor in spina-bifida and other malformations of the foetus. Foods rich in folic acid should be eaten before conception and after, especially in the first weeks of pregnancy, so that there is a sufficient level circulating in those vital first stages of the embryo development – the time when there is the greatest risk of abnormalities occurring in the division of cells. Mothers who have been on the pill before pregnancy, and those who have had several children in close proximity, have particularly high needs of a good folic acid level. Some wheatgerm daily is ample, but a good mnemonic is 'folic, folate, foliage' – thus dark green vegetables! Cook them very lightly for, like Vitamin C, folic acid is destroyed by boiling (keep the vegetable water for soups and sauces).

Vitamin E is thought to be helpful during the labour itself, so a diet rich in it – wheatgerm, vegetable oils and peanuts! – is good as a preparation. Vitamin K is needed for the clotting of blood – essential in childbirth – and a new baby will have low levels. Dark green vegetables like cabbage, sprouts and spinach are the best sources.

Minerals. There are about twenty minerals necessary for the human body, and the principal among them are calcium, phosphorus, magnesium, potassium and iron. These latter are essential rather than just advisable, and obviously they have a particular relevance dentally as they are the foundation stones of good mineralisation of the teeth. One of the other most significant factors of a plentiful supply of minerals during pregnancy is that it can confer a future resistance to tooth decay. Experiments have been carried out with two groups of genetically identical animal parents. One group of parents was given an unrefined 'good' diet, the other group a refined 'poor' diet; the resultant offspring were both fed on exactly the same diet as each other, and the offspring of the parents who had had the good diet developed tooth decay much more slowly. Somewhere along the line the mother had conferred a better resistance to tooth decay during pregnancy even though the babies were exposed after birth to the same environmental situation.

Calcium is obviously the king dentally, and a diet rich in this is vital during calcification (from the fourth week of pregnancy onwards, see page 28). Phosphorus is used in the formation of teeth and bones, and too high a proportion in relation to calcium – the ideal ratio is one to one – can cause maternal leg cramps, and tetany or muscular spasms in the first days of the baby's life. This can be controlled easily by eating less meat. Magnesium is present in bones, and there is a greater need for it in pregnancy. It is found plentifully in vegetables. Potassium has a close relationship with sodium or common salt, and if large amounts of salt are eaten, the ideal potassium/sodium ratio is upset. Salt is bad for us generally, and in pregnancy can cause a tendency to fluid retention and high blood pressure. Get used to eating your food without salt at this stage: its absence will be invaluable later and throughout life.

Iron has already been mentioned briefly, but a good intake is necessary. It is not easily absorbed, but Vitamin C helps. Iron can be depleted by taking the contraceptive pill, another reason for finding an alternative method of birth control for at least three months prior to conception. Iron is important for a number of reasons: it enhances and is enhanced by folic acid; it is also a factor in the avoidance of maternal anaemia. As the baby takes iron from his mother, needing sufficient reserves to carry him through the first months (there is little iron in breast milk; that in milk formulae is less well absorbed), problems can occur with prematurity, when too small a reserve has been built up in the baby.

Trace elements. These are present in the body and needed in relation to the action of minerals and vitamins. Zinc, found widely in food that has been raised or grown on zinc-rich soils, is needed for bones, and a deficiency can be the cause of stretch marks in pregnancy; iodine, found mainly in seafood, is vital to the proper functioning of the thyroid gland, and low levels in pregnancy can affect the intelligence of the child; manganese activates enzymes needed for normal skeletal development and thus plays an important role during pregnancy (it is available in many vegetables); and fluorine I shall discuss later.

The above are all the basic constituents of a good diet, but *balance* must be remembered. If a mother chooses fresh and good vegetables and fruit, keeps her meat intake low, and cuts out all processed or refined foods, sugars and salt completely, her health and that of her baby will be assured.

MATERNAL TEETH DURING PREGNANCY
The old wives' tale that every pregnancy costs a tooth, that the growing baby deprives a mother of minerals, thus weakening her teeth, is not entirely true. During pregnancy there are major upheavals in the body generally, and in the hormone levels, and it is the latter which affect the gums, giving rise to what is called pregnancy gingivitis. It is this that can weaken teeth indirectly, but I will discuss gum disease in detail in Chapter Seven: suffice to say here that if nutrition is poor – with a deficiency of calcium or zinc, for instance – then any disease process already present in the mouth will be magnified.

One of the other difficulties encountered at this time concerns pregnancy nausea or sickness and tooth decay. The advice given by many authorities is to eat small but frequent meals in order to avert nausea. Dentally, however, this can cause tooth decay, for it is the frequency of, say, sugar that is much more damaging than the quantity. On a good diet, most mothers wouldn't be taking much sugar anyway, but a good precaution during the nine months would be to brush after every meal, however small (this will also help to keep any gum disease at bay). If the nausea actually causes vomiting, the acid from the stomach can also start an erosion on the surface of the teeth. So, although it may be the last thing a nauseous mother wants to do, a good toothbrushing thereafter can prevent many problems.

DANGERS IN PREGNANCY
Ironically, a number of the major dangers during pregnancy can involve the dentist.

X-rays. It is because of dental X-rays that dentists must know about a patient's pregnancy. The dangers of X-rays at this time are an absolutely basic part of dental training, and although dental doses are tiny in comparison to those used on the body generally, they should not be given. For X-rays are a potent source of changes in the genetic structure and cell structure of any living mechanism. In fact, in a similar situation, I wonder if any research has been done on the effects a proximity to microwave ovens can have on a developing child. The effects, for instance, of VDUs on female workers have been highlighted recently: headaches and aching eyes were the least of them, too many miscarriages for comfort were apparently the worst. More research is very definitely needed in this field, because environmentally we are surrounded by too many factors which could, like X-rays, affect genetic as well as growing structures.

Mercury. The placenta, previously thought of as a barrier to prevent toxic substances reaching the baby, is in reality a membrane through which both good and bad substances of all sorts can pass. And one of the 'baddies' is mercury, a major constituent of the amalgam used in dental fillings. Mercury, described in greater detail in Chapter Nine, is undeniably a poisonous element, and any amalgam filling work can release a vapour which, however slight, can concentrate in the foetus. Given this fact, that we *know* mercury can cause problems even if it's in the smallest amounts, we want to reduce that amount to the barest minimum. The only answer is *not* to do fillings at all during pregnancy and during lactation, as mercury can pass into breast milk as well. It's a temptation for a mother *and* for a dentist to get old or new filling work done at the same time as the gum problem is being sorted out, but it's hazardous. Dentists should do routine scalings, give nutritional advice and advice on cleaning – the latter a major factor in controlling gum problems – but never any fillings if they can possibly avoid it.

Lead. Another heavy metal hazard is lead, which has been shown to concentrate, like mercury, in the foetus. I feel that pregnant mothers really ought to minimize the travelling they do in cars while there is still lead in petrol – and Britain is one of the few countries still to allow it. Any mother who lives near a major road, or in the centre of an industrial town or city, should be aware of the possible effects of that undeniable pollution upon her unborn child. This is where an organization like Foresight can play such an important part, doing tests to check levels of toxins in general. The hair analysis is particularly effective here: although the hair is dead, it was formed from general body tissues, and it can show three months of accumulation, whether vitamin, mineral or toxin. Holistically speaking, this is one of the best tests to perform as, primarily, it is non-invasive – it does not interfere with the body in any way – and it is also uniquely informative.

Lead and other toxins can also be taken in through the skin as well as the nose and mouth. Hands should be washed well before preparing food; fruit and vegetables bought or grown in industrial areas should be washed well; all chemicals that might be inhaled – and this includes spirit-based paints, and lots of gardening products – should be completely avoided during pregnancy.

Drugs. Anything and everything should be avoided during pregnancy, and ever since the thalidomide tragedy, the medical profession and the public have been all too aware of the effects drugs can have on the foetus. As mentioned in the section on pre-conceptual care, any drug-taking for a long-term condition will have been discussed previously with a doctor and possibly modified. But it's not only oral drugs that can harm: many creams or ointments for external use, those for eczema for example, are potentially hazardous if used or administered by an expectant mother.

The horrific effects the tetracyclines can have on calcifying teeth have already been discussed (page 26); and all patent remedies for colds, indigestion, nausea and other minor ailments should also be avoided.

Coffee, tea, cocoa, chocolate and cola drinks all contain the drug caffeine, and they ought to be cut out of the maternal diet. Herbal teas and pure juices could be substituted. Tea also contains fluoride which can have an effect on the bones and teeth of the growing child. Conscientious mothers often believe that by taking fluoride tablets during pregnancy they are helping their baby's teeth: there is in fact no conclusive proof that this does help, or indeed does harm, but as fluoride interferes with calcium – substitutes *for* calcium on teeth – the effects on the calcium content of bones seem to be very much more worrying. To come back to tea, some mothers drink up to twenty cups of tea a day: if they are also using fluoridated water, and perhaps taking tablets, they could be ingesting far too much fluoride, which could have a deleterious effect on their baby.

Smoking. Nicotine is a drug as well, and it plus the carbon monoxide in the blood of a smoking mother will pass into the baby's bloodstream. This can starve him of oxygen, resulting in poor development. Babies born to smoking mothers often appear – although full-term – as much as a month premature at birth. Poor body growth as well as poor intellectual growth are the results. Smoking is a major evil for unborn children, and must be avoided at all costs.

Alcohol. Large amounts of alcohol will harm a baby in the womb, and the baby is particularly vulnerable to such damage in the first eight to twelve weeks of development – another pointer to the necessity of cutting it out *before* conception to allow for the first few weeks of uncertainty as to whether conception has taken place. Alcohol will pass through the placenta, and in later months it is believed to affect the development of the foetal brain.

Food additives. These are the bane of modern diet, and something against which every holistic practitioner battles – and every other medical practitioner should. For commercial reasons only – for ease of manufacture, for customer temptation, for a longer shelf-life – colourings, anti-oxidants, flavourings, preservatives etc. are added to foods: few are nutrients; indeed few do us any good; some even rob the foods of what basic nutritional value they had. For they are often *chemicals*, and if we are beginning to realize that they can cause harm to grown bodies, the effect that they could have on *growing* bodies is too disturbing to contemplate. Again, in Britain, we seem to have been slower in cutting out many of these additives, thus many of the foods on sale here are looked upon as unsafe, even poisonous, in other countries. Avoid processed or refined foods whenever possible – a piece of advice that has cropped up before and will again. Baking a potato in the oven is just as easy, if more lengthy, than adding water to dried potato granules; preparing a green vegetable and steaming it for a few minutes is really no more time- or energy-consuming than opening a freezer packer or a can – and it's so much healthier. Not really enough is known as yet about the effects of additives on the body in general, nor on the developing foetus. To cut out all risks, cut out all foods containing additives.

Post-Natal Care

Right from the moment the new baby draws breath, there are many dental significances. And the first one, literally, involves that first breath. As we will see when discussing the fascinating oral environment, the mouth – as indeed does the body generally – nurtures a vast variety of bacteria, some benign, some not nearly so pleasant. If we can presume that at the moment of birth the baby's mouth was free of bacteria, as soon as he leaves the womb and is exposed to the atmosphere, he can breathe in and absorb bacteria and many other factors existing in the air, even in the supposedly sterile delivery room. These bacteria will form the basis of the baby's own unique oral environment, and can dictate whether or not he might ultimately be vulnerable to tooth decay.

However, less speculatively, at birth the baby's toothless gums will be holding within them some 44 teeth: the 20 baby or deciduous teeth with, above or below them, in the upper and lower jaws, the germs of 24 of the permanent teeth. All, at this stage, as already described, are at some vital stage of development. If the birth is prolonged, or causes stress to the baby, this can show up on the permanent teeth when they start to erupt 5–8 years later. If the tooth or teeth were being calcified at the time of birth (see page 25), then there will be signs of this, the neo-natal line, sometimes only visible to the professional's eyes, sometimes really quite obvious. Other factors which could disturb the teeth at birth are prematurity and haemalytic anaemia or jaundice. A prema-ture baby may be born without reserves of certain vital minerals such as calcium and iron which obviously will affect the teeth; indeed the prematurity may have been *caused* to some extent by some deficiency in the normal growth of the child. Babies who are born too soon will probably have to be kept in incubation, given drips, fed artificially, etc., and all this trauma could affect the tooth formation that will be going on at this time. A baby born with jaundice – due to an incompatibility of the cells of baby and mother – can lead to a colour staining of the chronological hyperplasia, the neo-natal line.

BREAST-FEEDING

A mother who breast-feeds her baby is giving him the very best possible start in life. Provided the mother is continuing the good, sensible and nourishing diet she ate while the baby was growing in the womb, her milk is perfectly formulated for her baby. It contains all the protein, vitamins, calcium and other minerals in absolutely the right proportions for her baby's total and correct nutrition, and man cannot improve on it. The colostrum which comes through in the first few days, a sticky yellow substance which precedes the milk proper, contains many antibodies from the mother that will protect the baby from a number of the infections and illnesses that could cause bodily and dental prob-lems; it is also very high in Vitamin A which is important for teeth. Enzymes in unheated milk – breast milk – help with hardening of the bones and of teeth; the protein molecules in breast milk are considerably smaller than those contained in cows' milk, and therefore protein and calcium are absorbed much more successfully. Altogether, it has been said that breast milk can mean fewer infections, fewer allergic diseases, less coeliac disease, fewer cot deaths, less future obesity and heart disease.

Holistically, from a nutritional point of view, I would recommend breast-feeding only, and for at least four months. However, it is undeniable that some mothers just cannot breast feed, whether because of illness or merely because they cannot seem to produce enough milk. (Sometimes, astoundingly, breast-feeding is avoided because of a supposed social inconvenience.) In all cases, if at all possible, I would hope that mothers would persevere – and be *encouraged* to persevere, for in some maternity hospitals, if there is difficulty, a baby is immediately put on to the bottle and on to formula cows' milk (it probably saves valuable nursing time). Even if breast-feeding cannot be continued, the mother should at least give the baby the colostrum of the first five or so days which is so rich in protective factors.

The classic phrase that nutritionists quote in this context is: 'Mother's milk is perfect for babies; cow's milk is perfect for calves.' Cows' milk, however modified for milk powders, *is* very much more concentrated in almost everything – which is not so surprising when you consider that a calf will grow from its birth weight to about 500–600 lb (225–270 kg) in its first year! Although some milk formulae are fairly well balanced – and are being improved all the time – they are *not* the natural food for babies. Millions of babies appear to thrive on them, of course, but I would rather see a return to the most natural form of baby feeding, that from the breast.

The other major advantage of breast-feeding your baby is that it gives a better jaw and mouth development. Many dentists and dental specialists have reported that they see fewer problems of jaw and tooth development in breast-fed babies. One book, in fact, quotes that in a survey of some 500 children with jaw problems requiring orthodontic work, only two had been breast-fed. The principal cause is thought to be the unnatural action of the muscles of the mouth and tongue that are brought into play when a baby sucks from a bottle. Often teat holes on a bottle are too large which means that the milk can gush down a baby's throat, depriving him therefore of his most basic desire, to suck. In general, sucking from a bottle is easier than from the breast, which is obviously a contributory factor as well. And as sucking is such a natural instinct, and the nipple is the natural thing to suck upon, any other action – such as that on the bottle teat – could with justification be termed abnormal. Bottle-fed babies can exhibit several types of malocclusion or crookedness of the teeth, which will probably require orthodontic treatment in the future. A new teat has been developed recently, however, which imitates the action of the nipple, and which, it is hoped, will reduce this tendency to malocclusion in bottle-fed babies.

The last – although certainly not the least – advantage of feeding from the breast is the undoubted greater intimacy between mother and child. Although babies who are bottle fed are held in the same position, and will probably receive as many cuddles and kisses, a closer relationship does seem to develop in breast-feeding. It is obviously difficult to prove in any scientific way, but it is perhaps due to the fact that a breast-fed baby who cries will be picked up, comforted *and* fed, probably, as well; a bottle-fed baby may have to wait for that feeding comfort until the correct feeding time, or at least until the bottle is prepared. As a result – and these inter-relationships and bases for the future *do* formulate this early – the breast-fed baby can grow up very much more secure in his mother's love.

Maternal diet during lactation. As during pregnancy, the needs for essentials are higher, and milk production can drain a breast-feeding mother as much as can the demands of the growing baby in the womb. A good diet will ensure that the milk is of good quality and that the mother's health is maintained. Foods rich in the B vitamins will help counteract tiredness and stress; frequent small meals might be more useful and palatable than three larger ones (although remember to clean the teeth well afterwards). The mother should drink a good quantity of liquid every day to ensure a good milk supply.

Many of the factors which affect the baby while in the womb can still affect him by passing through the milk. Dental work should still be avoided because of the mercury dangers; alcohol and many drugs such as aspirin, laxatives, sedatives etc., can enter the milk; smoking can reduce the milk supply; antibiotics, particularly the tetracyclines, can affect the baby; returning to the contraceptive pill can reduce milk supply slightly.

If the mother is careful at this stage in every way, if she is well fed and the baby is well fed too as a result, the likelihood of contracting any infection is substantially reduced: for it is in these first few months that many babies develop the colds, snuffles and feverish illnesses that can have so drastic an effect on the teeth. There is absolutely no doubt that there is a relationship between diet and good resistance to disease, whether bodily or dental.

TEETHING

The first thing to be said is that, despite all the risks and insults that can afflict a new baby – biochemical, dietary and genetic – it's really quite a tribute to the composition of human beings that most babies are born normally, grow normally, and their teeth grow relatively normally as well. Baby teeth, in fact, seem to be the least affected in every sense.

The chart on page 24 shows the approximate order and timing of the appearance of the baby or deciduous teeth. However, the timing is only a rough guide as many babies can remain toothless until they are at least one year old! The timing mechanisms are part of the baby's own individual blueprint, perhaps part of a pattern that he has inherited, and the teeth will come through when they are good and ready. Teething usually starts, though, when the baby is about 6 months, and all the deciduous teeth are usually through by the age of 2½ (the chart also shows the chronology of eruption of root and crown completion and calcification).

The baby is born with the baby teeth already formed in the gums. No one quite knows what causes them to erupt: it may be that the periodontal fibres grow and stretch, pushing the teeth out through the gums. However, we do know that the teething process can be painful to the baby – and to his parents!

The first signs of teething may be a reddish gum, a bump showing on the gum, dribbling, red patches on the cheek, or grizzling. Some babies are affected by all this, some are not. In general though, it is an uncomfortable time for the gums do become a little sore – not surprising, with the hardest substance in the body pushing through them. To ease this, I cannot recommend any of the topical reliefs available from chemists that you rub on the baby's gums: they are not particularly effective for one thing, and you will also be introducing the baby to drugs and chemicals of which we do not know the long-term effects, and some of the gel or powder (one brand used to contain mercury!) is likely to be swallowed. The same applies to the pain-relieving syrups which are swallowed: these are drugs too, and many of them are chock-full of sugar which is bad both dentally and from the point of view that you are perhaps familiarizing a baby with a sweet taste.

Cuddles and comfort would be a major relieving factor, with a clean finger perhaps rubbed on the sore gum; at least this will assure a grumpy baby that you're aware of the problem and that you care. Cold teething rings or hard chewing sticks can help; but a ring should only be fridge cold (not freezer cold which can 'burn' the gums and lips), and anything the baby is to put in his mouth must be scrupulously clean and safe (large enough so that it cannot be swallowed, and strong enough that no part can fracture off).

Teething is often associated with red bottoms or an increase in nappy rash. Teething isn't an infection which could perhaps exhibit in the urine or faeces and thus on the bottom skin; but it is an inflammation of sorts and, although the relationship isn't entirely clear, what is happening in the mouth can and does seem to repeat itself on the bottom. Scrupulous cleaning and frequent nappy changing will help prevent the problem from becoming worse.

Teething is used as a convenient scapegoat for almost everything; it's blamed for irritability, diarrhoea, loss of appetite, fevers and sickness. In reality, however, *none* of these are related at all to teething, except perhaps the first, and if a baby does seem to go off his food, the doctor must be consulted. Babies *do* get grizzly with the discomforts of teething, but they should still be *hungry*, should still need food, their most basic requirement.

As soon as the baby teeth erupt, they must be kept clean. Most experts advise the mother to clean around the tooth or teeth and gums with a small piece of clean gauze or a cotton-wool bud.

Some suggest using a little toothpaste on the gauze or cloth, but I would not advise this as toothpastes, even 'natural' ones, are quite chemically strong, and some is bound to be swallowed. Many baby toothpastes contain sugar, and most toothpastes contain fluoride; the latter will be of variable value as, although the topical or direct effect on the baby teeth will be protective (although baby teeth do not seem to take up fluoride as much as permanent), the value of swallowing anything containing fluoride is much more debatable. It's not necessarily the toothpaste that cleans anyway, it's the massage and rubbing, and I'll discuss that in Chapter Eight. A very soft toothbrush can be used later – perhaps with the merest suggestion of toothpaste – which will help accustom the child to brushing and indeed when he is allowed to hold and use the brush himself, it can become a pleasurable game.

MOVING ON FROM BREAST MILK ALONE

Breast-feeding should be carried on as long as possible, and unless there's a very good reason for it, mothers shouldn't feel that there's a great rush to move their babies on to mixed feeding. In the recent past there was a lot of pressure on parents to start this process early, within the first three months (often for commercial, occasionally for medical, reasons), but ideas, thankfully, have now changed. Breast milk is all that is needed for *at least* the first four months, and it can be carried on longer, for up to six to eight months alone, especially when the baby's parents suffer from allergies – eczema, asthma, hayfever etc. – and the baby might be vulnerable as well as a result. A baby introduced to foods other than milk at an early stage will suck less at the breast: the breasts will therefore get less stimulation, and will produce less milk; and the baby will ultimately not get *enough* milk. This obviously has significance nutritionally for it is milk which is the optimum food for growth at this stage; and the lack of sucking will also affect the jaws. And a baby's digestive system is not capable, until at least three months old, of absorbing foods more complex than milk.

Often a mother can feel instinctively when her baby is ready to start trying something other than milk. If he seems restless and hungry *before* four months, he should be allowed to suck longer at each feed, or he could be fed more frequently throughout the day. Only in exceptional cases should this be read as the signal that he wants to move on to other foods. But if *after* four months he shows the same symptoms, he may be ready: other signs are when his birth weight has doubled, or when weight increase has slowed down considerably. By about six months, though, the baby definitely does need more nutrients than milk alone can supply – although milk from the breast can and should still remain a valuable part of the diet for as long as the mother wishes to continue feeding.

Check carefully after each new introduction of food to see that it does not have an adverse effect – causing diarrhoea for instance – and try only one food at a time, so that if there is a reaction, the food can be pinpointed accurately and immediately.

Juices. The first things to try are juices – from about four to five months – and therefore perhaps one of the first investments for your baby's health ought to be the price of a juice extractor. Don't just think of the citrus fruits with their high content of Vitamin C; juiced cauliflower, cabbage, turnip and green beans also contain C in good amounts, as well as a variety of other goodnesses such as calcium. Carrot, the traditional 'first' vegetable for babies, contains a very digestible form of calcium as well as Vitamin A, and can easily be juiced. Most of the vitamins of vegetables and fruit are contained near the skin, but all have to be peeled or at least washed and scraped as it is the skin that is the fibrous part of the plant. The baby's digestive system could not cope with that – and another consideration is that the vegetable or fruit might have been sprayed (do try to buy organic and unsprayed products at all times). All juices must be diluted with cooled, boiled filtered water for their nutrients are too concentrated at this stage, and start with 1 teaspoon a day. Just because a baby seems to like carrot juice, say, don't give it to him daily for the next week. That may bore him, and anyway it's fun for him and for you to try a wide variety of tastes – as long as basic precautions are taken. Try peach or mango, apple or tomato (sieve to ensure there is no skin or pips). Do be wary, though, for some citrus fruits and strawberries can cause allergies. When you start experimenting with juices, you can be very inventive.

If you can't afford to buy a juice extractor, chopped vegetables can be puréed with some cooled boiled water in an electric liquidiser or food processor. When puréed, strain through a fine mesh sieve to retain any fibrous material. Don't *heat* juices as this will destroy many of the vitamins.

The one thing to absolutely avoid is commercial fruit juices, especially those made with babies in mind, because they're still, astonishingly, made with a sweet syrup base. Stick to pure unadulterated fruit and vegetable juices with no additives or preservatives. I'm not even entirely happy about carton juices which are designated pure (and indeed have no additives or preservatives): they have been conditioned or heated, which takes *away*, I think, from their nutritional value – but they're all right to use as a standby.

Purées. The next phase of mixed infant feeding is the sloppy purées which require little or no chewing. These should be introduced slowly, with only 1 teaspoon being offered at one meal (at lunchtime for example, when the baby is not as frantic with hunger as he is in the morning). The texture should be fairly wet and soft at first, thinned down with breast milk or boiled, cooled, filtered water.

All the many baby books around give lots of ideas of the best foods to serve as purées – and those to avoid. Things like ripe bananas, carrots, apples or pears are good first foods. Cooking, of course, takes away some of the vitamins, but apples and carrots do really have to be lightly cooked before mashing or puréeing. A food offered at body temperature instead of stone cold, will probably be accepted more easily anyway. Heat very slightly so that the chill is taken off. Another excellent fruit, rich in Vitamin E and unsaturated fatty acids, is the avocado pear which mashes down easily like banana.

Many experts say that a cereal is a good first purée type food, but beware, as there is a small possibility of coeliac disease (gluten allergy) from wheat cereals such as wholemeal porridge, semolina etc. Other wholegrain cereals could be too high in fibre for a baby: these could have a locking-up effect on the calcium as well as zinc and magnesium. (Remember to avoid the calcium-robbing foods such as rhubarb and spinach as well.) Many baby cereals have added vitamins which sound beneficial, but along with all the vitamins in the natural food, plus possible supplements, a baby could in fact be getting *too much*. One of the better cereals in terms of allergies, for instance, is baby rice – but it too has had this and that added to it, and I really would prefer to see a more natural vitamin intake in fresh fruits and vegetables only.

In West Germany, organic baby foods are on sale, but as usual we are quite a way behind in Britain. Many of our dried baby foods, jars and cans are, sad to say, added to, coloured, sugared and salted, although they are getting better, and they should only be used in emergencies. It's appropriate to mention here, too, that mothers should always look at the labels of baby foods if they must buy them. It will be a salutary lesson to see how much is added, or how much the foods are 'modified'; and it must always be remembered that the ingredients are listed in diminishing quantity order: if water is first – quite common – it means that there is more water than anything else!

But one of the very best foods at this stage must be the sprouts of seeds and pulses. Many things can be sprouted – soya beans, chick peas, fenugreek seeds, lentils, buckwheat – and the sprouts which enrich so many Chinese dishes are those of the Mung bean. Sprouts are easy to grow at home, are cheap – 1 lb (450 g) seeds or beans can be grown to make 7–10 lb (3–4.5 kg) of sprouts! – they are absolutely free of allergens and pollutants, and are rich in nutrients for everyone, particularly babies. They contain virtually the whole range of vitamins and very easily digestible protein. The proteins that are inside the seed or pulse are converted in the sprouting process to amino acids, which are the constituents of protein; thus half the digestive process has already been undertaken by the actual sprouting process itself. In order to visualize more clearly the nutrients that are locked up and then released by sprouting, consider the simple sunflower seed: think of its size and then the size of the plant which grows from it. All the potential for that growth is contained within one tiny seed!

The best seed for babies is probably alfalfa, the smallest seed and sprout. Put a handful of seeds in a large clean glass jar, and cover with water. Leave to soak for an hour or so, then cover the top of the jar with muslin or a piece of J-cloth held on with an elastic band. Drain the water away through the cloth, and put the jar into a dry dark place. Repeat the soaking and draining procedure once a day and the sprouts should be ready in about

3–4 days. When ready, remove from the jar and place them in a bowl of cold water. Stir around to free the husks – the fibrous part – which should float to the surface and can be tipped away. Cut away any remaining husks, and purée the root and the sprout, moistening them with a little cooled boiled water or breast milk.

Solid foods. This is really a misnomer, for 'solid' foods should not really be considered in terms of a baby until the chewing molars are present (the firsts come in at about 12–16 months, and the seconds at 1¾–2½ years). But that chewing reflex is there, and as the baby gets older and will eat more, and his digestive system becomes more sophisticated, he can cope with rougher, thicker textures which could more justifiably be termed 'solid' foods. Many babies are put on to solid foods far too quickly because it is thought they need to get their jaws working properly. Their jaws are already working quite adequately, and a new choice and texture of foods is really only relevant from the point of view that the baby has an increased choice of nutrients.

When moving on from purées, do so gradually. Use 1 teaspoon of diced foods, say, to half a cup of puréed foods to get a texture that will be acceptable. The diced foods must be soft – no fibrous meat at this stage – for it is the gums that will be doing most of the chewing work. Keep an eye on how the foods are being digested: if the baby is spitting them out, getting tummy pains or the food is passing through in chunks, the baby may not be quite ready for this texture stage yet. The digestive system may not be mature, or the baby isn't managing to chew the food enough in the mouth first (for chewing and saliva are major initial stages of proper and full digestion, see the next chapter).

Never forget about finger foods which are good for gums and for teething. In the earlier stages there are dangers of bits flaking off some finger foods and causing the baby to choke, but most finger foods will massage gums, clean tiny teeth once they erupt, and feed the baby well at the same time. Try peeled, quartered and cored apple, peeled raw carrots, fingers of peeled cucumber and other vegetables, and baked crusts of wholemeal bread.

At some time within this first year – at about eight months usually – many babies are weaned off the breast (or the bottle), and on to doorstep cows' milk. I have already mentioned my misgivings about cows' milk for young babies – its concentration in so many factors, particularly sodium – and I feel that the emphasis put by so many child nutritionists on the milk content of a child's diet is perhaps over-stated. It's the calcium, the vitamins and minerals that are considered vital, but all of these can come from a good sensible wholefood diet, thus cutting out the necessity for a huge intake of milk. This may be considered revolutionary by some, but cows' milk does contain sodium in excess, it does have protein in larger, therefore more indigestible, molecules, and it may well contain hormones, antibiotics and stabilizers. The pasteurization process itself renders the calcium content of the milk less soluble, and raw unpasteurized milk or goats' milk – both rarely available – would be better. (The latter in fact is lower in sodium than cows' milk, and it may help to reduce allergic problems.)

However, the basic point is that once the baby is off the breast or bottle, it is not entirely necessary for him to continue drinking milk. If he is on a good diet, with lots of sprouts, vegetable and fruit purées etc., he will be getting enough calcium and other essentials.

One of the milk products of which I approve is yoghurt, and this can be useful from the very earliest mixed feeding stages onwards. For those who feel I may be contradicting the norm, flying in the face of accepted thinking, yoghurt is, of course, milk, but it is milk that is converted into a much more soluble form of calcium by the yoghurt bacteria. It should be live and natural, and is best made at home. Fruit can be added to it to make a change, and that is far more nourishing and satisfactory than commercial fruit yoghurts which can have up to 1 tablespoon sugar in them!

The transition from breast milk to no milk, if you choose to do this, should be slow, however, and yoghurt will be a good substitute along with all the other infant foods already specified.

Eating with the family. Once the baby is past the stage of transition – he has got all his baby teeth and is eating and enjoying a wide range of good foods – he will be able to join in with family meals. In fact the earlier he can do this the better: he can learn that eating in company is enjoyable, which could help to prevent eating problems later, and of course it's all part of his learning process. But it must be remembered that babies are brighter than most people think: if they're regularly eating their nutritious sprouts but a sibling or father is tucking into chops and chips, they'll soon feel that they're missing out on something. Many conscientious parents do tend to feed their baby on the best possible foods, preparing it with the utmost care, while carrying on the same bad dietary habits themselves. There's a lot to be said for the whole family changing its eating habits at this stage, or even earlier perhaps, so that the baby's ultimate health – as well as that of the rest of the family – can be ensured.

Children from about two onwards have different growth phases, have differing appetites, and this is an age when many eating problems occur. Parental example is a major influence – if you eat and enjoy your lightly cooked greens, the chances are the baby will too – but it may just be that the baby isn't very hungry, because he's going through a quiescent period of growth. And, just because a baby or child won't eat, don't cram him full of sugars because you think that anything – a favourite pudding, say – is better than nothing. In general, puddings aren't very good nutritionally, but of course if you have only yoghurt or fruit available, these could be light and enjoyable, and fruit will quench a thirst as well as feed.

For those that eat meat, it should be introduced in small amounts at first, but it should always be obtained from trustworthy sources if at all possible: ensure that no growth promoters or hormones have been used to make the animals put on weight; and that the butchery and hanging have been carried out in the old traditional ways which will give best flavour and quality. Many holistic and wholefood nutritionists are against meat in general, and advocate alternative protein sources, but I believe meat can be all right as long as in smallish quantities, for it is undoubtedly rich in good proteins for babies, as well as many of the fats that they need. Try to avoid the richer redder meats such as beef and lamb (avoid pork altogether), and serve poultry instead. (Fish of course is as good a source of protein and other essentials.) Liver too is nutritious, and a good source of Vitamin K and iron.

When cooking for the family and the baby, remember that a baby needn't grow up with a yearning or taste for highly seasoned foods. His taste buds will not relish foods with sugar and salt –

which are bad for us all – as long as he is never introduced to them. Try to get used to omitting them from cooking if you can: if not, season at the end of cooking a meal to be shared by a baby, *after* taking out the baby's portion. A basic dietary rule to remember at this stage in the baby's life – and thereafter if possible – is that foods in general should be as natural as possible, as lightly cooked as possible, and for a more detailed résumé of the 'recipe' for good diet and health, see Chapter Ten.

DECIDUOUS TEETH AND THE DENTIST

Holistic dentists would like to be involved with children's teeth right from the very beginning, and obviously this depends to a very large extent on the parent and his or her relationship with the dentist. We would hope, as already mentioned, to have given advice before conception and during pregnancy, but often it happens that a mother is so involved *after* the pregnancy – and there is a quite natural reluctance to bring a screaming baby into the dental surgery! – that she will not consult the dentist again for some six months. This lost time, as far as her own dental health is concerned, could be alarming, but it is also a time when the dentist could be contributing a great deal to the future dental health of her child. He can help with teething problems, continue his dietary advice, and become aware of any potential problems as the child's teeth develop. When a new parent comes into the dental surgery for a check-up or treatment at regular intervals, the child should be brought along too.

This can alleviate all sorts of worries on all sides. The baby and toddler will gradually become accustomed to the man in the white coat and will become familiar with the smells of a dental surgery (all images that have been retained with horror in the minds of those who had early traumas concerning teeth and the dentist). The parents too will be able to gain reassurance in all aspects of their child's teeth that might be worrying them.

Deciduous abnormalities. Baby teeth usually grow without any problems at all, and the most common worry is about timing. If a neighbour's baby has got all its front teeth, and yours is still grinning toothlessly, don't think that he is backward: the teeth do just take their own time.

If a parent is worried about the position of a child's teeth as they erupt – if they don't sit centrally on the gum ridge, say – the dentist can also reassure. This is where the action of the lips and the tongue will come into play. Even if the baby teeth are not in the correct position when they erupt, the lips, tongue and cheeks will soon push them into a nice arc.

It is also important that the dentist can look at the jaw size and shape, and the spacing of the teeth of a baby and child. It's not unusual, for instance, that the upper jaw sticks out more than the lower jaw in baby dentition: this does not necessarily mean that they'll have that slightly goofy look to the permanent teeth – although genetics too will play their part. If nutrition has been good throughout pregnancy and afterwards, the jaw will be given the potential to be wide, allowing good spacing between the teeth. But genetic factors here too should be taken into consideration, and a mother who had crowded baby teeth and then required orthodontic extractions or whatever on her permanent teeth, may have passed this on to her child. Crowded baby teeth almost always mean crowded permanent teeth, and this needs careful monitoring right from the very beginning because with crowding comes an inevitable vulnerability to tooth decay. A parent at this stage and in this situation should have detailed advice from the dentist on diet so that foods which will cause decay – sugars and refined carbohydrates – can be assiduously avoided, and advice on cleaning, which will be more difficult if the teeth are tight and the brush filaments cannot get between them.

Baby teeth are obviously important for function and growth, but parents don't need generally to worry about the odd strange thing happening. This will not necessarily mean that the permanent teeth are going to have the same problems because, surprisingly, there's not often a very close relationship between the two sets of teeth.

Tooth decay on deciduous teeth. But where the relationship *does* matter is when there is tooth decay. Although the deciduous teeth are shed, and aren't therefore permanent, any decay can be much more serious than many parents realize. If decay is allowed to set in, the deciduous teeth, which are slightly softer than the permanent, may be lost. As part of their function is to keep a space open in the jaw for the permanent teeth, any loss of tooth will mean the gap may be closed, therefore permanent teeth may grow more crookedly or tightly together. It is vital that baby teeth are looked after well, and it is the sole responsibility of the parent to monitor diet and cleaning for at least the whole deciduous period – and indeed throughout the whole period of mixed dentition which comes next, up to about the age of nine or ten.

The major villains of the piece at this stage are sugars, and sweet-eating should always be discouraged. Children's drinks, too, although often advertized as being full of Vitamin C, are so full of sugar that any benefits are thereby nullified. Pure fruit or vegetable juices, heavily diluted sugar-free juices or just plain water are all that are needed, and indeed if a child is eating a good nourishing wholefood diet, he won't be all that thirsty anyhow. Another horrifying contributory factor in baby tooth decay is the habit – hopefully now becoming rarer – of coating a baby's dummy with a syrupy drink or honey as a pacifier. It may temporarily placate a screaming baby or toddler, but the ensuing traumas when tooth decay occurs and dental treatments are necessary, would seem to far outweigh any such short-lived peace.

And this is one of the major considerations when attempting to avoid deciduous tooth decay. A child with decay will have to go to the dentist for treatment; a child with decay will have to undergo drilling, filling, fear and discomfort. No dentist wishes to inflict this upon anyone, especially a toddler; no parent should allow a child to reach this stage. A child of three or four will not have the patience to stay in a dental chair for longer than a few minutes, so treatment can often be difficult anyway; and any discomfort experienced now could have a permanent effect on the child and his perception of the dentist in years to come. The dentist, too, experiences problems when he encounters baby tooth decay. He would like to build up a relationship with his patients in an advisory, caring sense, talking about such problems as crowding and staining; he does not want to have to drill and fill, to perform what is in effect destructive treatment, and to treat a disease which could have been prevented.

This is indeed why holistic dentists believe emphatically in prevention starting before birth and continuing meticulously through the years. Children who experience dental traumas – and I consider anything more than just a quick look and probe at the teeth a trauma – are likely to react badly to the dentist and therefore to the care of their teeth in the future. There is inevitable child variation, of course, with some children perfectly happy to accept treatment (dependent on good parental attitudes and a good considerate dentist to a large extent), but on average, no one, neither child nor adult, finds any sort of dental treatment pleasant, and therefore prevention should be of paramount importance from the very beginning.

One major aspect of prevention at this deciduous stage is considered to be the use of fluoride drops and fluoride tablets. Fluoride is undoubtedly effective against tooth decay, but holistic practitioners feel that there is no way in which the amount of fluoride being ingested can be accurately gauged. With fluoride in some water supplies, fluoride in toothpastes, fluoride occurring naturally in some foods, then ingestion may be too great and staining of teeth can occur. More potentially serious, though, in these first six years or so of life and growth, is the effect the fluoride might have on the growing bones and tissues of the body. Fluoride has an effect on calcifying tissue, and the formative materials that are being used for growth and hardness are not only forming teeth, but are forming bones as well. If fluoride is being ingested in large amounts, what effect is that having on the growing bones of a child? The answer is that no one really knows, and this is the holistic argument against fluoride: if the effect on the body of any substance is not exactly or accurately known, then it should not be ingested by the body. To be honest, in my heart of hearts, and from a balanced reading of arguments both for and against, I am an agnostic: I know the undoubted dental benefits of fluoride, but not knowing the long-term effects of drops or tablets taken in these first few growing years, I could not possibly advocate their use. This is *not* because I believe it's wrong, but basically because I just do not know.

Topical fluoride can be useful though at this stage: it is painted directly on to the tooth enamel where it can do good without having any effect on the rest of the body. However, it is not safe to use on too young a child, as a baby will not be able to prevent itself swallowing.

Again, to take a holistic approach, if the diet is good enough, then the teeth should be safe from decay without the additional help of fluoride. The use of fluoride assumes that the teeth *will* decay, therefore aims to make them harder and more resistant, treating the effects and not the cause; but by good diet, from a sound nutritional base which started before the baby was born, we could claim that a child will not develop tooth decay anyway.

Thumb-sucking and other habits. Sucking is such a basic instinct for a baby that it can start in the womb: scans have shown the near-term baby sucking a thumb or finger. Associated in the earliest days with the pleasure of feeding, thereafter it can be a comfort at times of stress, hunger or tiredness. A thumb-sucker isn't a deficient child, one who is lacking love or basic caring: it's just a little habit that, provided it stops at the right age, will not be particularly harmful. Up to the age of about seven it should not be too actively discouraged – the comfort value often outweighs the potential damage to the jaws – but it should never be actively encouraged either.

But after this age, it ought to be stopped for, with the remodelling of the jaw during the next eruption phase, that of the permanent teeth, the pressure of the thumb and the sucking action can lead to a severe class 2 appearance – the upper jaw obtrusive, the lower jaw pushed back – which will require extensive orthodontic work. (It could also lead to later TMJ problems, see Chapter Ten.) The holistic dentist can advise on ways in which a child can be weaned off thumb-sucking: indeed an orthodontic appliance is often the answer, as thumb-sucking and a plate just do not go together.

The way in which children suck their thumb or fingers can occasionally cause the teeth to take on funny shapes, where they have been depressed or worn away by the constant repetitive action. They can wear away right up to the gumline, often showing a sort of halo effect. For baby teeth are not as durable in terms of wear and tear as the permanent teeth, and once the enamel has been breached, the underlying dentine is relatively soft and can wear away fairly quickly. Grinding the teeth can bring about similar effects.

Dental advice here ought to be that it is nothing really to worry about, the teeth are not permanent, and this will not affect the permanent teeth waiting to come in – as long as care is taken and potentially damaging habits are stopped in time.

Accidental damage to a baby tooth. When a baby starts to walk, he is unsteady and can easily fall over; thereafter up to the period of mixed dentition, at about six, he is exploring his world, and has little fear. It is a time when many accidents can happen, and luckily nature has compensated for this in a number of ways. Dentally, the jaw bone is more flexible, allowing for bumps and bangs that a more mature jaw could not take; the baby teeth too are protected in that they can sustain a much greater degree of damage than can the permanent teeth. Often a baby tooth can be quite severely displaced during a fall, but within a couple of days can be pushed back into its previous position by the action of the tongue and cheeks. Generally, the pulps of baby teeth are well supplied with blood vessels, nerves etc., and the apical foramen is often quite large where the tooth joins the bone and where all the nerves and blood vessels flow from the bone into the tooth. When a baby tooth is banged, there is often a bruising – the tooth will actually look grey or black – but within a couple of weeks this coloration gradually disappears and the tooth will liven up and become white again. This is because of the good supply of blood inside the tooth which washes away the bruised tissue and allows new healthy nerve endings and blood supply to be replaced inside the tooth. This doesn't always happen, of course, and the tooth could die if the damage were too great, when there might be a little dental abscess, a gumboil, occurring above the tooth. The same damaging bang to a permanent tooth, to compare, would nearly always cause the death of the tooth. Once there has been internal bleeding and inflammation, the pressure build-up inside the nerve chamber is so great that it constricts any further blood supply coming into the tooth and so the tooth dies.

Care During the Mixed Dentition Period

In baby dentition, the full arc of twenty teeth will normally be complete by 2½ years. We then have a period of rest dentally until about six when there are often the first signs of eruption of the first permanent molars. With the arrival of these teeth, we enter the era of what is called mixed dentition, when the jaw contains both baby teeth and permanent teeth.

FROM BABY TEETH TO PERMANENT TEETH

This is the beginning of a time of continual change which goes on for years: from six to eight, a lot is happening; from eight to ten, there's normally a lull; and then from ten to twelve, there is a great deal of activity again. This is 'teething' in a real sense, filling the mouth with teeth which will be those utilized for a lifetime, and it can cause discomfort in the early stages – although it's ironic that no one ever attributes a six-year-old's moods to teething!

From the ages of six to twelve, a small mouth can often look a hotch-potch, with gaps, half-grown teeth, and what sometimes looks like double or treble rows of teeth. If the jaw is wide enough and grows well and normally throughout this period everything should sort itself out. In the western world, however, due to both dietary and genetic problems, there are undeniable problems, and thus orthodontic treatment is often necessary.

The body in general during this time is undertaking periods of growth, usually in spurts, and thus it is too with the teeth. As with the eruption of the deciduous baby teeth, the timing of the loss of baby teeth and the eruption of permanent teeth is all a matter of individual body or genetic patterns, and there are no definitive rules. The first are usually the molars at the back, between six and eight years, and then there is a loss of the lower incisors followed by the lower laterals. Next are the upper central and lateral incisors. When this has been attained, normally by 8½, there is a period of rest and there is no further loss of teeth until the child is about ten years old. This is when the lower baby canines fall out to be replaced by the permanent canines. The other permanent teeth all erupt during the next few years, until about thirteen, excluding the third molars which generally erupt from about seventeen to twenty-one. These timings are not always related to these ages because growth hormones could possibly play a part too: the spurts in general growth associated with both boys and girls at the very onset of puberty could coincide with spurts in tooth growth as well, and it's not uncommon for children of fourteen or fifteen to still have some baby teeth which, on average, would have gone from the mouth at about twelve. The chart on page 25 shows the approximate chronology of permanent tooth gain.

The first permanent teeth to come in, usually the first molars, don't actually take the place of any of the other baby teeth, but come up further behind or at the back of the last baby molars, the Es. This eruption can be accompanied by some discomfort as these teeth are large – the largest of our molars – and the gum flap that covers them can be quite tough for the tooth to break through. Sometimes there can be what we call an eruption cyst and this is where the tissue above the tooth fills with fluid and forms a little lump in the mouth. This can look quite alarming – often a blue-black ball – but it's comparatively painless and the child can usually burst it by simply biting into it with the opposing teeth. If parents get alarmed, the dentist can quickly lance it, if necessary, and the tooth will then erupt quite normally on its own.

Sometimes, though, there isn't a permanent tooth behind or underneath the baby tooth, in which case a baby tooth – usually an E, the last of the baby molars, or the C, the baby canine – can remain in place. Thus it's not uncommon to see adults of twenty to twenty-five, even up to the age of forty, still with a baby tooth retained in place, and it's often left there for cosmetic reasons (there'd be a gap otherwise). This would seem to suggest, although we don't fully understand the mechanisms of eruption, that it is the stimulus of the permanent teeth underneath that makes the baby teeth fall out.

Another contributory factor is the activity of the cells already mentioned, the osteoclasts and osteoblasts, which work assiduously through periods of growth, eating and forming bone. To use the baby Es as an example again: there are often three roots on a baby E, and the permanent tooth above or below – if it's there, and if it's in the right position – will fit snugly into the hollow created by the baby roots. As the permanent tooth grows, the osteoclasts will eat the baby roots, the permanent tooth will move further up into the inverted U-shape, and the baby tooth, loosened by its diminishing root structure, will start to wobble and will eventually come out. This is when children can work the loose tooth with their tongues (many *adults* still talk about the pleasures of inserting a tongue into the side of a loose baby tooth to encourage it on its way), and this 'helping hand' is no bad thing: a loose tooth present for too long can mean bacteria and trapped food debris. But it should not be encouraged when a tooth has hardly any mobility; many children can be over-enthusiastic about baby teeth loss, thinking about the coin left under the pillow by the fairies (although this is a useful way of making the loss and changeover of teeth into a happy and interesting event, both for parent and for child).

Sometimes, though, when permanent teeth erupt to the side of baby teeth – giving the appearance of a double row or banking of teeth – the baby teeth can take a little longer to fall out. In extreme cases, when they are very stubborn, and are preventing the permanent tooth from moving into its correct position, a dentist may need to give that final push, perhaps even by extraction (the one time the removal of a baby tooth by 'unnatural' means could be beneficial). The permanent tooth will then move into its designated place by the action of tongue and cheeks. Sometimes indeed, a permanent tooth can come through earlier than expected, when a baby tooth is missing because of accident or extraction, and the permanent tooth hasn't got the opposition of dissolving away the baby root.

Throughout this whole period, when the activity is so high, cleaning the teeth properly is difficult and must be scrupulously overseen by parents. There are irregularities not just in the position of the teeth, but also in the height of the teeth, with some baby teeth being pushed and tilted by the permanent teeth underneath. With the added hazards of loose teeth and some inevitable crowding, it is a time when children are most vulnerable to tooth decay and dental infections. It is also a time when sweet-eating might be at its height: even if parents have scrupulously avoided sweet things at home, once children start school, they'll inevitably encounter them. Avoidance of sugars and rigorous cleaning will be the answers here, as well as topical fluoride which will be soaked up by the more porous enamel of the new teeth and give protection.

But altogether, the whole process of transition from baby teeth to permanent teeth is a remarkable one: it's usually very rapid in biological terms, and it all goes astonishingly smoothly considering all the things that can go wrong. The mouth and jaw at this time are in constant turmoil, in a constant state of activity, and in the main children seem to cope, and there does seem to be a normal and predictable pattern. However, things can and do go wrong, and this is probably where the orthodontist steps in.

PLANNING ORTHODONTICS

Orthodontics and mixed dentition automatically go together and are inextricably linked. Through orthodontic awareness at an early age a dentist can plan in advance, and obviate many potentially distressing problems. A good dentist, hand in glove with a caring parent, will have been enabled to see the development of his youthful patient; will be monitoring general growth in tandem with growth of jaws; will know if bottle-feeding or thumb-sucking is likely to lead to malocclusion; and will be overseeing the transition from deciduous to permanent teeth. A conscientious dentist – not necessarily holistic – should start planning orthodontically as soon as any potential problem first reveals itself.

The study and practice of orthodontics – which, formally, is the regulation or straightening of teeth – is still expanding, and has become a very important part of progressive – and preventative – dentistry. Although I believe that diet plays a major role in ensuring that jaw and teeth form to their maximum potential, in an imperfect world, orthodontics is becoming increasingly relevant. For by having good straight teeth through orthodontic planning and treatment, the patient will be happier with his appearance and will thus, hopefully, pay more attention to his teeth in the future; if teeth are straight and not too tightly crammed together, they will be easier to clean. If toothbrush filaments and floss can easily reach in between teeth, bacteria will not gather, therefore the likelihood of disease on gums and between the teeth is dramatically diminished. These, plus the way the teeth and jaws function, are the major factors governing prevention through orthodontics.

Orthodontic treatment can entail the use of appliances such as braces, and it may also require the extraction of teeth. It all depends on the individual mouth of the child, and by keeping a close watch on developments the good dentist – who will either initiate the orthodontic plan himself, or do so in tandem with a specialist orthodontist – can fairly accurately predict what will happen in terms of jaw expansion, growth of bone in the jaw, size of teeth and potential crowding. To get the full orthodontic picture, however, X-rays may need to be taken. Although holistically I am reluctant to consider radiation in relation to growing tissue and bones, this is a time when it may be vital. The dentist will be able to see the size, position and angle of the jaws and the situation of the permanent teeth, see if there are too many or too few, and plan accordingly. A new and promising development in orthodontic treatments is the potential for *expanding* the jaw, as opposed to diminishing it by extraction.

Most orthodontic treatment does not start until the child is about eleven or twelve. It can be started earlier, but this of course involves the removal of baby teeth which I am not in favour of unless absolutely necessary. It can also involve what we call serial extractions when, perhaps, several baby teeth are removed at the sides to make the front four teeth look better. This may help temporarily, but it doesn't really *alleviate* the orthodontic problem, and will mean more extraction when the permanent teeth come in. Serial extractions were popular some years ago, but many consultant orthodontists now have different views, thinking more about the psychology of the child than of the ideal textbook orthodontic situation. For a child who has perhaps been very dentally fit, and who is faced with extractions at seven to eight, followed by more at eleven or twelve, will not have very positive ideas about treatment at the dentist, and may become reluctant to wear a brace.

Parents *ought* to be concerned as their children's teeth grow, and should never be frightened to ask for advice from their dentist, especially when the child is in the eight to ten age group. Planning, followed by treatment at about eleven or twelve, is best. If orthodontic treatment is left until the child is fourteen, say, the child may be reluctant to have his appearance marred by a brace, and could indeed be subject to ridicule from his peers. To have treatment at about twelve, along with a majority of his friends, would probably make him feel much less alone. And getting the teeth right at this stage – treatment which is available to all now, both on the National Health Service and privately – will ensure good dentition for the rest of the child's life, with a good appearance and less disease. If older children and teenagers – and indeed adults – feel that a lot of time and trouble (and sometimes money) has been spent in correcting the teeth, then all of them should, hopefully, be very much more interested in looking after their teeth in the future – the ultimate prevention.

COLOUR OF TEETH

Teeth come in shades of all colours, almost literally, but white is rare, believe it or not. Dentists who have to make crowns are required to match colours of teeth, and they use shade guides relying on, in dental terms, many separate colour variations. The most common shades are of grey, yellow, brown or — yes — orange! Using these four as a basis, with variations and tints on each, most people fit into these categories.

The actual colour of a tooth depends very much on the thickness of the tooth: if it is thin, the tooth will have a more translucent appearance and will often appear more grey. Indeed if you look closely, as a dentist has to do in order to match shades for crowns, shades of blue or pink can show through due to the translucency of the tooth.

And it is at the mixed dentition stage that parents begin to feel worried about the colour of their children's teeth. When, for instance, a child has got two new permanent front teeth, they can look very discoloured — yellow or grey, say — in comparison with the baby teeth: these do often look whiter because they're smaller and because of the amount of calcium of which they're composed. Parents can be reassured in that once all the permanent teeth are through, the colour will look uniform and good.

Other colour fears could indeed be justified due to a tetracycline prescribed during pregnancy or infancy, or to fluorosis. A tooth which is greyer in colour than others, whether deciduous or permanent, could be due to tooth death after a bang. And the new front permanent teeth often have areas of hypo-calcification when little spots, blotches or stripes of colour, usually white, are clearly visible. These may become less conspicuous as the other teeth come in, in that they will all look uniform, but the imperfections may be permanent, due perhaps to abnormalities of nutrition of the tooth at a crucial early stage.

TRANSPLANTING TEETH

Just as the two- to six-year-old stage is fairly adventurous, so are the later stages when children seem never to have any fear or take any care. This is a time when a permanent tooth may be knocked out and this is much more serious. If the child can be rushed to the dentist with the tooth kept moist, then often the tooth can be replanted by the dentist. This will tend to be a more surgical operation than a simple re-insertion in the hope that nerves might regenerate. The latter has been known to happen, but a lasting success is rare. With the advances of current science, however, when severed arms have been sewn back on successfully, the future possibilities of cell growth and stimulation cannot be entirely dismissed. Currently, dentists are relying on a process similar to root filling, and this sort of transplantation can work reasonably well for up to ten years. A permanent tooth that is knocked out is a pity, but it need not be a permanent disaster, and indeed can occasionally be the basis of a new, improved and less destructive orthodontic plan: why take out *more* sound teeth when an accident has already deprived the mouth of one.

Permanent Teeth

Although many adults nowadays may have crooked or crowded teeth, our children can now have perfect jaws, teeth and dental arches because of good nutrition, good hygiene, caring dentistry and efficient orthodontic treatment. That the latter may depend on a couple of years of minor discomfort and a minimally less than exciting appearance if a brace is worn, should never be allowed to matter, for the future of the teeth that are needed for the rest of life is at stake. Parents can still play a supportive and encouraging role at this stage, and indeed the teenage years – when children may perhaps 'revolt' to a certain extent – can be very destructive to the teeth. For this is a time when diet can be very poor indeed – fizzy drinks, fast foods, biscuits, sugary snacks and cakes to assuage the hungers that assail teenagers – and as a result these are the years when tooth decay can set in. Most people who require dental fillings in their twenties and thirties will have laid the foundations of that decay when in their teens.

Although it may be difficult for parents to make their voices heard, they should try to help still, in a number of ways. A continuing good diet at home will help to offset the new dietary temptations that present themselves when teenagers have money of their own; an early dental hygiene regime will, hopefully, carry on as habit with the teenager; encouragement to go to the dentist regularly will be another major factor in prevention.

WISDOM TEETH

These are the last of our permanent teeth, and they can influence the dentition from about the age of sixteen, although they may not erupt until the later teens or early twenties: in fact I knew someone who was seventy before his erupted! Historically, wisdom teeth were the 'reserves'. When primitive man wore down his teeth by chewing and grinding on abrasive foods, in effect the teeth grew smaller and moved forwards – in what we call the mesial drift – which we think may be nature's way of allowing room for the reserves to grow into the mouth. Today, we lack abrasive foods, our teeth don't wear down, and yet there's still the mesial drift to allow for the wisdom teeth. Both the mesial drift and the teeth themselves can cause problems.

The mesial drift occurs even without wisdom teeth, and this can affect orthodontic treatment. If at the age of fifteen, the teeth have been orthodontically persuaded into a lovely straight arch, then the mesial drift can undo all that work, making the teeth tight together again, even overlapping sometimes. The potential of this should always be monitored by the dentist very carefully, because it would be a shame to have a wonderfully aesthetic result at fifteen which developed into a mess at twenty.

The wisdom teeth are almost superfluous to our needs nowadays, and jaws have become smaller anyway. The usual answer is extraction both from the orthodontic point of view, and also because they can undoubtedly cause problems. They can erupt in a bad position – jammed against the tooth in front, or into the bone, or indeed into the tissue and muscle at the end of the gum ridge – because there isn't room for them. This pressure can cause pain in itself, but there could also be a space between the wisdom tooth and the swollen gum in which food and bacteria could collect, which can often cause inflammation and pain. Any wisdom teeth will, probably, as a result, have to be removed. To call them wisdom teeth is a misnomer nowadays, anyway, for it is anything but wise to have them!

CHAPTER FOUR

The Fascinating World of the Mouth

The mouth is probably the hardest-working organ of the whole body. It is almost constantly in use – when we swallow, talk, eat, drink, chew and kiss – and it is a unique environment. The mouth acts as a major funnel through which most influences and substances are introduced into the body, and thus it has to cope with irritants of all kinds to a far greater degree than any other part of the body: it is an extremely hardy place, and is constantly in turmoil.

The mouth is fed all the time, adapting to hot and cold substances, to the rough surfaces of food, to introduced chemicals perhaps, and it is in the mouth, on the tongue, that one of the body senses is situated, that of taste. The mouth is the start of the alimentary system and prepares food and drink so that it is acceptable to the rest of the body: the lips will test first then accept and close around a food or drink; cold substances are warmed, hot substances are cooled; chunks of food bitten off by the incisors are then chewed and minced by the molars to a consistency acceptable to the digestive tract and system. The mouth is also intimately associated with breathing.

Despite all these differing procedures and potential hazards, it is rarely that the mouth will be damaged: only occasionally does a hot food actually burn; even more occasionally does a sharp edge on a food tear the tissue. In fact the mouth contains rows of the hardest element in the body – the teeth – and very infrequently does damage occur to the mouth tissue from that source. The mouth is even immune apparently to many allergic reactions.

Nickel, for instance, is a common allergen, and one patient who wore nickel earrings had an allergic reaction around her ear. When the earrings were removed, the rash disappeared. Later, however, the patient was fitted with a dental appliance containing nickel, and the allergic reaction returned – but on her *ear*, not in her mouth!

The mouth, therefore, has unique properties because of its function as a funnel into the rest of the body, and is an extraordinarily complex organ. The saliva which is produced by glands in the mouth plays a major part in the ecology and biochemistry of the mouth, and indeed of the digestion: it is in a sense the lubricating oil which keeps the mouth going. If the body is healthy and the saliva is therefore rich in the right elements, saliva can help prevent tooth decay and gum disease – although, it can also *contribute* to dental disease.

For the mouth, along with the rest of the body, is home to millions upon millions of bacteria – although it's not an image many people like to conjure up. Many are benign, many are malign, but in the right conditions a good healthy balance can be maintained. In the wrong conditions (wrong for us, right for them), these bacteria can make the mouth into a bit of a cess-pit. They feed on the food – especially carbohydrates – passing through the mouth; they settle themselves comfortably in crevices on the teeth out of the way of disturbances from toothbrush or floss; they swill around in the mouth in the saliva, moving from one part of the mouth to another; they can contribute to bad tastes and to bad breath; and it is these bacteria – along with the saliva in its less beneficial aspects – that form plaque, the major causative factor in both tooth decay and gum disease.

Saliva and its Functions

Saliva – common or garden spit – is a very complex, useful and fundamental part of our system. Indeed saliva marks the start of the digestive system, the one that keeps us all going in the sense that we couldn't live without food, and properly digested food at that.

There are three major pairs of saliva glands in the mouth: the largest, the parotids, lie in the cheek tissue just below and in front of the ear, with ducts issuing into the mouth near the upper back teeth. The two smaller pairs lie under the tongue (the sub-lingual) and the lower jaw (the sub-mandibular); their ducts empty below the tongue. (The location of these larger glands is relevant in dentistry because they are associated with the build-up of hard calculus or tartar, most common on the back of the front bottom incisors and on the cheek side of the back molars.) There are also a host of other, very small saliva-producing glands lining the cheeks.

The production of saliva is controlled by the sympathetic and para-sympathetic nerve systems, which partially explains an increased salivary flow when we're stressed or excited, and a decreased salivary flow – a dry mouth – when we're frightened. The glands are most stimulated when food is in the mouth – that's their major job – and they are often *over*-stimulated by sharper or more acid foods or drinks. In fasting periods, overnight, say, the saliva flow is diminished.

Each one of us produces a different type of saliva, dependent on the health of the body, and what we're eating: but salivas are also different from person to person in terms of flow, viscosity and composition. The average hourly flow of saliva is about 20 millilitres (just over ½ fluid ounce) but it can vary from a resting flow of 0.5 ml (too small to convert) to 111 ml (about 4 fluid ounces) hourly. The more the glands are used, the more saliva they tend to produce, so someone who is eating and drinking a lot throughout the day, and indeed throughout the night, could theoretically be producing – and probably swallowing – just under 2¾ litres (4¾ pints) of saliva daily! An *average* daily flow is, of course, a little more modest – about 450 ml or ¾ pint. Significantly, if there is a shortfall in saliva – when the glands produce less than average or necessary – there is an immediate increase in the bacteria in the mouth (they're multiplying, but not being swallowed down), and there can be severe recession of the gums. Dentists will immediately notice a rise in tooth decay if saliva flow has been reduced by, say, illness, by irradiation of the face (when saliva glands are killed), or other conditions such as mumps which affect the parotids. Saliva production can be diminished by the menopause, and by age, although the latter may be more related to the poorer health of older people in general. In fact, people who suffer congenitally from dry mouths, or whose saliva glands have been affected by illness, are often given artificial saliva, a solution which they swill around in their mouths. It seems to me, holistically, that it would be better to investigate thoroughly the *causes* of the salivary dysfunction instead of treating the effect. However, any encouragement of saliva is good in that it increases the resistance to tooth decay.

The different saliva glands in the mouth have different viscosities, some thicker and more sticky than others: the runnier the better, apparently! The composition of saliva – cells, enzymes, salts, minerals and proteins that are circulating in the body generally (although it's 99.4 per cent water) – can vary from person to person, even if they are on the same diet, due to the inherent differences in their individual biochemistry. The variations in flow, thickness and content of saliva are relevant because upon them can depend the amount of gum disease or tooth decay that might be produced.

Below is a listing of the various functions of saliva. They are not in any significant order, but will merely reveal a little of the complexity of an extremely underrated product of the body.

Digestion. This, as already mentioned, is the major function of saliva, and it changes from youth to age: the baby saliva glands which form at about six months (another reason for a lot of dribbling then) contain enzymes to help in the digestion of milk; older saliva glands contain enzymes which will help break down more complex foods such as starches.

Saliva production is intimately associated with digestion and with all the senses associated with food. The classic experiment is that of Pavlov's dogs who began to salivate when a bell rang because they had been conditioned to believe the bell meant food. Similarly, we produce more saliva when hungry or when expecting to eat, and the sense of smell – that most neglected of our senses – also plays an important part here. Smelling and seeing food in preparation, even associating sounds like cutlery being laid on a table with the imminent arrival of food, can make our mouths water in anticipation. And by the very act of doing so, the body is beginning the act of digestion even before a morsel of food has reached the mouth.

Taste. You must have saliva to taste, for although the taste receptors are separate from the saliva glands, they only function when foods are in solution, in a liquid environment. They cannot work if a food is bone dry, and you can test this yourself by touching a dry biscuit with the tip of your tongue, or by placing a piece of biscuit on the tongue. Only when you start to moisturize with saliva does the taste come through.

Lubrication. Saliva is a lubricant, enabling hard things like biscuits to be softened. When you chew, the food is combined with saliva into boluses, or balls, which can slosh around in the mouth and thus can be swallowed easily. Lack of chewing and therefore less saliva can mean difficulty in swallowing – the Victorian precept of chewing everything at least ten or twenty times was a biologically sensible one – and it can lead to digestive problems.

Barrier effect. In association with lubrication, the saliva acts as a barrier to protect the mucosa or tissues from harmful substances. The oily mucousy film produced on cheek tissues, for instance, will act as a slide over which potentially damaging foods can pass easily: a dry mouth is very much more vulnerable to damage.

Buffering effect. Saliva helps to buffer or protect the mouth from, say, acid or alkaline foods or conditions in the mouth. If a food is acid, it can have a corrosive effect on the tooth enamel, and indeed can cause a reaction in the mouth generally: think of the exaggerated reactions of those who bite into a lemon. When this happens, the saliva glands go into top gear, and are stimulated to produce more saliva in order to dilute and reduce the acidic effect. The saliva also contains chemicals in it which help neutralize the effects of too much acidity or alkalinity. The buffering effect has been found to work most efficiently at mealtimes; proteins and vegetables increase the effect, carbohydrates decrease it.

Anti-bacterial effect. Saliva contains many of the antibodies and antigens that are found generally in the bloodstream, and which help in the fight against disease. Enzymes in saliva have also been shown to slow up the growth of the bacteria in the mouth. All these are important in relation to the control of dental disease because the proper composition of the saliva – dependent in turn on a healthy body in general – will mean more or less disease.

Blood-clotting effect. This is one of the most 'magical' functions of saliva, and one of the most commonly used – if least appreciated. Animals lick their wounds for this very reason, as indeed do we instinctively. Saliva on a cut helps stop the blood flow, and probably has an element of the anti-bacterial effect as well. This is more clearly seen, of course, in wounds to the mouth: a cut lip or the gaping hole after extraction of a tooth stop bleeding and heal very much more quickly than would any other part of the body.

Water balance. The saliva glands will tell the body when more water is needed. In conditions of dehydration, the glands will produce less saliva, so the body needs to drink in order to feel more comfortable. Even a dry throat will enable /the mind to register that the body is thirsty and needs more water.

Excretion. As saliva contains certain elements like minerals which are in the body generally, so it can contain traces of heavy metals like lead or mercury. There's so much activity in all the little blood vessels feeding the saliva that anything in the blood supply will obviously pass through. The amount of this excretion into the saliva is very small – much less than the kidneys, say, which are the main excretory organs for the body 'rubbish' – but it could be used as a method of detection for toxins that might be in the body. It's not an excretion in any real sense, though, in that it's ingested again by the body, being resorbed, and passed backwards and forwards. Spitting would be a truer way of excretion, but that is not only anti-social, it can be dangerous. For, as the saliva contains body bacteria, so it can contain viruses and diseases such as TB, rabies (the classic disease associated with spit and foaming at the mouth), hepatitis, herpes, polio, AIDS, etc. With many of these diseases, it is the body fluid, the spit, that can be the contagious element. Disease, therefore, can be transmitted by saliva.

Remineralization of teeth. Saliva contains many of the minerals circulating in the body, particularly calcium, and thus saliva can actively be instrumental in putting minerals *back* into a tooth. Tooth decay means a demineralization of the tooth to a large extent – when the mineral content of a tooth has been breached and is under attack – but often enamel can merely be dissolved fractionally by acidic foods or drinks. The calcium content of the saliva will deposit on the tooth and remineralize it: even the beginnings of a tooth decay cavity can be halted, reversed even, by the calcium deposition from healthy saliva.

Too much calcium in the saliva, however, can contribute to tooth decay because, oddly, the plaque bacteria revel in lots of calcium, and too much calcium can also form into little stone-like deposits in the saliva ducts.

Growth factor. A final function attributed to saliva by many researchers – but not scientifically proved – is that it can stimulate growth of skin and nerves. This could easily be so because of its undoubted abilities to promote rapid clotting and healing of tissue: if a nerve is severed in the mouth, the saliva could well promote cell regrowth in tandem with its other qualities. Even skin lesions will show rapid regrowth with no scarring in a very short space of time. Altogether, the mouth has a remarkable power to heal quickly after damage. At the risk of repetition, it is a priority of nature, because if the mouth were not in functional order, the body could die.

BAD BREATH

One of the less beneficial aspects of saliva is its relation to bad breath, and this can be partially due to bacterial activity in the mouth as well. In some cases a bad breath can be caused by poor digestion in the stomach – noticeable when you burp – or it can be the result of emissions from the lungs, particularly obvious in smokers. Indeed garlic is exhaled from the lungs rather than from the stomach, and garlic and spices do actually penetrate the tissue of the mouth and the digestive tract: they are, after all, used to penetrate dead tissue – the meat that we eat – so they can leach into living tissue as well. (A particularly spicy or garlicky meal can result in *skin* and *sweat* leaching out these odours.) In most cases, though, it has been shown that bad breath is due almost entirely to conditions in the mouth.

The principal causative factors are stagnation of food debris and dead cells in the mouth – for, like skin, cells are continually being shed from the teeth, cheeks and tongue etc., and if they're not washed away by saliva, they will then putrefy in various nooks and crannies in the mouth. This is why in the morning – after a nocturnal diminishment in the flow of saliva – we wake up with dry, foul-tasting mouths and a bad breath. And slimmers, fasting in the cause of health and beauty, are horrified at the emissions from their mouths. This is also why older people tend to have bad breath, because the saliva flow reduces with age.

Another major cause of bad breath can be tissue destruction following either tooth decay or gum disease. A large hole in the tooth can harbour lots of bacteria, debris and putrefying tissue, and obviously unpleasant smells will be the result. An abscess could well smell, and a sufferer might be able to *taste* that as well. Gum disease has a characteristic smell all of its own, and most dentists can identify it immediately and differentiate the smell of even the mildest gum disease from that of a decaying tooth, stagnation of food, or the saliva.

Saliva itself is of a smelly nature anyway. It has been shown that if saliva is incubated for 1½ hours, it gives off smells characteristic of those identifiable in bad breath. This is again why it's important to have a good salivary flow, for it will be swallowed and not retained anti-socially in the mouth. Drinking and eating will help, both because of the washing-away effect of the food and drink, and because of the increased flow of saliva.

The most effective way of reducing bad breath is to brush the teeth. This will shift the stagnant debris which, along with bacteria and saliva, will be spat out. If toothpaste is used, there will be a pleasant taste and smell. Another way of reducing bad breath is by mouth rinsing, possibly with a commercial mouth-wash. Holistically, though, both toothpaste and mouthwashes contain chemicals which could possibly be doing as much damage as they are good in the sense that they will cause chemical upset in the mouth – they may kill off the wrong bacteria – and, to be honest, it is a little like masking the smell of sweat by applying a deodorant on top of the sweat. However, as a temporary relief from bad tastes and smells, they can be effective and, as both toothpastes and mouthwashes are swilled around and then spat out, they are not ingested to any great degree.

One of the most embarrassing aspects of bad breath is that, in most cases, the sufferer isn't aware of it. When we first become aware of a smell, it's very noticeable, but once that smell has been around for a while – we *keep* smelling it – the nerve receptors become saturated, and we are no longer aware of the smell. Thus it could be with your own bad breath, and it may indeed be a case of 'only your best friend will tell you'!

The gases given off by bad breath have been analysed, and the most predominant are hydrogen sulphide – with its characteristic rotten egg or cabbage smell – and diamethyl sulphide (which is ammonia-like). Bad breath has also been measured. By using liquid nitrogen, scientists have frozen bad breath; after warming it up again, they can measure the odour with an osmoscope. The bad breath can then be graded according to how much it needs to be diluted before the smell is completely neutralized. You could then be told *scientifically* just how bad your breath is.

However, as a last thought on breath, it could be sexually attractive! Breath is almost invariably thought of in relation to the word 'bad', but babies, for instance, have sweet breaths which mothers find irresistible. As skin is a well-known source of sexually stimulating smells, so too could be the breath, as both skin and the mouth have the same sort of secretions. The sense of smell, and the pheromones, are potent factors in sexual chemistry, and it could be that someone who is virile, attractive and *healthy*, could have a breath which is a stimulant to the opposite sex, especially someone who is known and sexually familiar.

Bacteria in the Mouth

That the human body is host and prey to millions of bacteria of some sort or another, is well known. There are bacteria in the air around us, bacteria on the skin, bacteria living in organs throughout the body, and bacteria within the mouth and on our breath. A baby in the womb has a sterile mouth as far as we know, but the minute he leaves the womb and is exposed to the environment, he acquires his own colonies of mouth bacteria and funguses which come to him via his mother, through the air of the room in which he first draws breath, and from the breath of those present – parents, doctor, midwife etc. As these mouth bacteria are so relevant to tooth decay – some are more destructive than others – one could almost claim that if the midwife, say, had a particularly virulent colony of streptococci in her mouth, she might be conferring on that new-born baby the potential for future tooth decay. In fact, in this mouth-bacteriological sense, there is almost an argument *against* having babies in hospitals, for so many more peculiar bacteria and funguses could be present in a hospital, however sterile, than in a more bacteriologically natural home environment.

These original colonies will, of course, be modified by later colonies obtained from food and environment, but it could be argued that by presenting the right bacteria to a new mouth – the ones that are thought to be least destructive – the vulnerability to tooth decay might be diminished. A lot of research has been and is being done into the various types of bacteria which cause tooth decay and gum disease, and indeed into the premise that if you *reduce* certain types, then that mouth is environmentally more secure against mouth disease. Holistically, I believe that life isn't that simple, nor indeed are the biochemistry and bacteriology of the mouth. I do feel, however, that the combinations of bacteria that are first formed in the mouth could certainly alter the resistance of the host.

However, from that first breath, the baby's mouth begins to foster its own bacteria. One researcher found twelve different kinds of bacteria within the first day; by the end of the first ten days, the number had increased to twenty-one. After eruption of the teeth, the bacterial content of a child's mouth is similar to an adult's, and, depending on how clean those mouths are kept, the total count of micro-organisms in the saliva in the mouth is of the order of hundreds of millions per millilitre. This means that the average person can swallow between 1 and 2.5 grams of bacteria per day – about three-quarters of a teaspoon. Or, to put it another

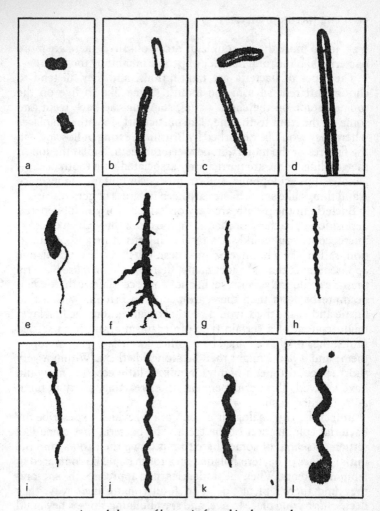

Actual shapes of bacteria found in the mouth

a. Cocci

b. Non-motile rods

c. Non-motile curved and fusiform rods

d. Part of a non-motile filamentous rod

e. Motile curved rod with flagella attached at mid-point of cell

f. Motile rod with peritrichous flagella

g.h. Small spirochaetes

i.j. Medium spirochaetes

k. Large spirochaete

l. Large spirochaete showing reproductive division

(Magnification approx. x 3000)

way, in no more than a couple of drops of saliva, there are more bacteria than the total number of people inhabiting the earth!

The types of bacteria are multifarious, and they all tend to choose different sites in the mouth. Some like to live on the tongue, some on the cheek tissue, some on the back teeth and some on the front teeth. They like particularly to gather in places where they won't be disturbed by brushing, eating or flossing – in the fissures of the molars, in between the teeth, and at the top of the gumline. Some are particularly associated with tooth decay – lactobacillus acidophilus, and streptococcus mutans, for instance – and things like spirochaetes are keen on areas of gum disease.

Bacteria in the mouth are very orderly, and if you looked at a deposition of bacteria or plaque on the tooth through an electron microscope, you would see a fascinating structure and organization, rather like a beehive or ants' nest. On that one tooth, in one apparent layer that is in fact many, there would be more bacteria than we could truly conceive: in one square centimetre there could be more bacteria than there are people in Britain. Within that hustle and bustle there would be total organization: the first layer might consist of a certain type of organism arranged in serried ranks; they might be joined by another cocci, say, lying on top of them; and a flagyl might then lie alongside them. Within a very short space of time, a highly organized little eco-system would have evolved, all inter-dependent, inter-reacting, a city in miniature or microcosm.

In fact the city analogy is a good one by which to describe the bacterial colonization of the teeth. The bacteria first come like settlers in search of somewhere to put down their roots, and the initial bulges of bacterial plaque on a tooth could be compared to temporary tents. When the settlers learn to appreciate the site, and they find there's plenty of good food coming their way, they decide it's a good place to live, and start building cities. They build across the tooth, covering every available surface. After a while, of course, it all becomes too crowded, and the bacteria cannot expand over the ground – or tooth – any further. The next direction in which to build is up – and bacterial expansion at this stage is very similar indeed to the conditions that led to the proliferation of skyscrapers in crowded inner cities. In fact there's so much going on in the mouth – and remember that what I described above is happening on *one tooth only* (multiply by at least thirty!) – that it's a wonder most people aren't kept awake at night with all the activity!

Saliva + Bacteria = Plaque

Despite all its beneficial aspects, it is the saliva that provides the basis upon which the bacteria grow and form plaque. Imagine a tooth that has been totally and thoroughly cleaned of all its surface layers so that there is only spotlessly clean and gleaming enamel: within twenty minutes of this in any mouth there is a deposition of a film containing some of the constituents of the saliva on the tooth's surface. The film is thin – known dentally as the acquired pellicle – but within that twenty minutes (sometimes even less), a layer of complex proteins, calcium and phosphates will have built up on that gleaming surface. This acts rather like a sticky flypaper, to which the bacteria are attracted, and upon which they can sustain a grip. They would find it very difficult to lie on the polished clean enamel, but the saliva film provides a textured surface upon which they can securely and comfortably settle.

There are several theories of how and why this pellicle forms, and the most rational would seem to be that the calcium in the saliva tends to concentrate on the tooth's surface – after all, the saliva does have this property of remineralization. It could be likened to the furring up of a kettle: as a kettle will form an inner surface concentration of elements in the water, so the teeth 'fur up' in the same way with the concentration of calcium. Indeed, experiments have shown that if saliva is dried on a glass slide, the same hard-to-remove calcium deposit occurs. And it would seem that the bacteria *like* these calcium deposits, and need them in order to form. All these factors in conjunction may be why there is such a quick colonization of the tooth's surface by this film matrix and then thereafter by the bacteria.

It seems strange that the body should produce this layer naturally when it seems, to all intents and purposes, to be potentially harmful to the body. And by going back to primitive people who had healthy diets and teeth, it seems that even then the layer was produced. It must have had some purpose in nature, and experiments have shown that the pellicle does seem to concentrate things like fluoride and trace minerals as well as the calcium, which would perhaps have protected the teeth from bacterial attack. The pellicle film could protect and lubricate, and it may be that only when it is modified, by a less than perfect diet, say (when health of the body and of the saliva are affected as well), that bacteria can proliferate enough to form the basis of disease. Tests on animals have tended to confirm that plaque formation is less rapid and virulent if the diet is of a wholefood and primitive nature, but only tests on human beings would have true scientific validity, and this would be extremely difficult to set up. An experiment based on a comparison between someone on a 'western' or 'rubbish' diet in strict nutritional terms, and someone on a primitive wholefood diet, to see if there was a difference in the formation and type of plaque produced, has not been undertaken to my knowledge – probably because of the comparative difficulties involved (individual biochemistry and resistance, the inevitable variances in environmental terms etc.). There might be *no* appreciable difference in the results, but I feel, holistically, that there would be, and this of course is what science is all about: it is a leap in the dark, and only after making an initial assumption and then by proving it, can it be turned into scientific fact.

THE FORMATION AND COMPOSITION OF PLAQUE

So, from a totally clean tooth surface to a tooth covered with a calcium-rich pellicle takes only a few minutes. The pellicle starts to form from the gum area and works its way up the tooth, and the bacteria too, within that same twenty minutes, collect, adhere to the pellicle, and work their way upwards similarly. After the initial colonization *along* the tooth's surface, the layer starts getting thicker. At the start the bacteria may only be a couple of microns thick (virtually immeasurable, for bacteria are *very* small), but within about twenty-four hours, say, you can have a reasonably thick layer – the skyscrapers of the city analogy – that can be seen with the naked eye, and that can be scraped off the tooth's surface with a fingernail. And that scraping, of a yellowish-white mush, is plaque, and it is a living entity. You might be looking, on one nail, at hundreds of millions of bacteria of many different species and all in some form of organization.

The bacteria in the upper layers of the plaque will be different from those in the lower layers, for they change with the thickness and age of the plaque. Cocci formations may have been the first to settle, for instance, but as the layer got thicker, there might be a predominance of another form or shape of bacteria. Also, with a thickening of the layer, the bacteria nearest the tooth's surface will have less oxygen so anaerobic bacteria – which do not need oxygen – will thereafter tend to flourish there.

The actual composition of plaque is very complex chemically. Apart from the myriad bacteria species, there could be funguses, food debris, proteins, living cells, dead cells, and other varying constituents of saliva. The superabundance in plaque is of calcium and phosphate though, which come from the saliva, and which would almost appear to have been pumped in! The cells and bacteria present in the plaque inter-react with each other; there is also an inter-reaction between the different species of bacteria; and there are enzyme reactions as well. The mouth in itself may be a busy place, but the activity in the plaque layer is terrifying!

As briefly mentioned, plaque differs from one part of the mouth to another. The plaque which lies closest to the gums is of a different composition because the gum surrounding a tooth actually secretes fluids of its own, which a certain type of bacteria likes. The plaque on the back teeth will be different from that on the front teeth, partially due to the influence of the parotid saliva glands. Another reason may be that foods can linger on the back teeth – they're more difficult to clean thoroughly – and thus a different type of plaque will take advantage of that.

THE PROPERTIES OF PLAQUE

The bacteria in plaque can produce acid, and can cause tissue destruction; this is why plaque is directly responsible for both tooth decay and gum disease.

It is the acid produced by plaque that eats into the calcium of the tooth (not the bacteria themselves) to cause the beginnings of decay. And this acid is produced on an intake of carbohydrate, mainly sucrose or ordinary white sugar. Plaque can produce acids from other sugars, even quite complex natural ones, but it has a very special relationship with sucrose, and seems to like it best of all. And it's a high sucrose intake – the sugar that we dentists scream about constantly – that produces the most acid and thus the most tooth decay.

Acidity and alkalinity levels in the mouth are measured on a pH scale which ranges from 0–14: 0–7 is acid, 7–14 is alkaline. (Skin is also measured on a pH scale: a dry skin can have its natural acidity restored by a skin tonic or even by a diluted application of vinegar.) The more acid the mouth becomes – through acid production from plaque, or actually from what we eat (acidic foods, like lemon) – the lower the pH value. The lower the pH, the more destructive the plaque acid will be on the tooth's surface. Eating too much citrus fruit – which is very acidic – can also act directly on the tooth's surface, even without the presence of plaque, and dissolve the calcium on the tooth. This is *not* tooth decay, however, and this loss of calcium can usually be restored by the remineralizing action of the saliva.

But with the intake of sucrose or similar sugars, and the consequent acid production of the plaque, the pH of saliva can drop within about two to three minutes to quite a low level. If someone had plaque on their teeth, and had some sugar in a meal, there could be acid on the teeth *within two minutes*. The rapidity of the whole process cannot be emphasized enough, and unless one got up in the middle of a meal to brush the teeth, there could, literally, be the beginnings of tooth decay. For this reason, and it does seem unlikely I admit, *it is much better to brush teeth before a meal rather than after*.

As plaque contains enzymes which can turn sugar into acid, so it contains enzymes which can cause tissue destruction. Incipient tooth decay can be caused by plaque acid within an hour at least; if plaque is left on the tooth's surface in the proximity to the gumline (where of course it starts), there can be a sufficient thickness or concentration after twenty-four hours to cause gingivitis which is an inflammation of the gum tissue, and the beginnings of gum disease. The plaque can eat the gum away – which is what causes the bleeding – and as it also contains enzymes which release ammonia, hydrogen sulphide and mercaptan – all of which are potential irritants – the condition can be magnified, and can contribute to bad breath as well. More significantly dentally, these toxins or irritants appear to initiate a reaction which makes the gum and bone shrink away from the tooth. It's the change in the alveolar bone that is the most worrying as there is a physical resorption and degeneration which means the tooth is held less securely and could be lost. Plaque also appears to produce a destruction of the periodontal fibres, the little suspension hammocks which hold the tooth into the bone, and this too means ultimate tooth loss.

Another property of plaque is that after it has ingested minerals from food and saliva, it can go hard – and this hard plaque is known as tartar or dental calculus. The calculus hardens on top of an active plaque layer, thus making it extremely difficult to get at the plaque to brush it off. The calculus layer itself is relatively inactive, and if it were polished it wouldn't cause problems; but it is naturally rough in texture, so can attract more plaque and bacteria to exacerbate any existing problems. It must be removed to prevent possible tissue damage from its roughness and in order to get at the plaque underneath, and this can only be adequately done by the dentist or hygienist.

Calculus can occur above or below the gumline, and thus is more of an influence in gum disease than in tooth decay. Supragingival calculus is when the calculus goes above the gumline, *on* the gum; sub-gingival calculus is the one that creeps up under the gum margin where it meets the tooth. Supra can often be seen, on the tongue side of the lower front teeth or on the cheek sides of the upper teeth – where the saliva glands emit – and it is often a yellow-brown colour. Sub can occur almost anywhere and is often green, brown or black: its formation is more to do with the gum fluids than with saliva. In severe build-up of calculus, whole teeth can be so covered that they lose their shape; the thickness can be about 12 mm (½ inch); and calculus can even form on dentures if they're not cleaned properly!

The quantity of calculus formation varies enormously from person to person, and it could be something to do with diet. Hard water can contribute to a greater build-up than soft, although this is a personal observation rather than scientific fact. Younger children suffer very little calculus deposit, but this can change as soon as they reach puberty, which suggests a hormonal influence. Stress, too, can contribute to a calculus build-up, and many dentists observe this on patients who attend regularly and whom they know well.

A plaque layer can be brushed off the teeth at home, but once calculus has formed, only the dentist or, preferably, the dental hygienist, can remove it. It needs to be 'hoiked' or scaled off with a metallic instrument; in some cases calculus can be vibrated off the tooth by using ultrasonic equipment. Calculus removal is a major function of dental hygienists, and indeed is one of the things that keeps them in work!

Plaque then, the almost inevitable product of the fascinating world of the mouth, is a major cause of both tooth decay and gum disease, and everyone – child, parent, patient, dentist and special-ist – should battle to eradicate it. Every mouth will probably always form plaque – and some more than others, for diet, heredity and individual resistance do play a significant part as well – but if it is properly controlled by good hygiene (see Chapter Eight), and by every other piece of armoury at man's disposal, dental disease could be diminished to a very high degree. We have to look for some way in which we can produce a good healthy body environment which will produce in turn a good mouth environment. Diet, it seems to me, is that system – the best, the safest, and the most sensible way of preventing dental disease.

CHAPTER FIVE

Tooth Decay

Although tooth decay is very rarely life threatening, it can be painful, very disfiguring, and extremely expensive. In Britain in 1982, something like 29½ million fillings were performed by dentists. If this seems outrageous already, that figure only includes treatments in England and Wales (for Scotland lists its figures separately); only those done on the National Health (it does not include those done privately, which will add a very considerable number); and the figure must also be seen in relation to the number of people who go to the dentist on a regular basis, which is well known to be no more than 50 per cent of the population. If we take all these factors into consideration, it can mean that there was one filling *at least* for every person that went to the dentist! These fillings were the result of tooth decay.

The cost to the National Health Service of treatments in 1982 was a staggering 536½ million pounds, and much of that would have been expended on tooth decay. That figure is only what it cost us as a nation, and did not include the cost of productive time lost by workers attending the dentist. To take the concept even further, that enormous but nominal cost does not include the valuable learning hours lost by schoolchildren, the equally valuable leisure hours lost by adults and children alike, nor indeed the hours which dentists could be utilizing much more effectively with dietary and hygiene instruction.

For all this money, time and discomfort is being expended on a disease which is entirely preventable: it is absolutely undeniable that by a combination of good diet, good hygiene techniques and fluoride therapy, tooth decay could be virtually eliminated. In fact, since 1982 when the above figures were recorded, it can truthfully be said that the levels of tooth decay in Britain have fallen, and some of this is due to the work of the local dental authorities, and, surprisingly, the toothpaste manufacturers. Not only have they included fluoride in their toothpastes, but they have instituted the publication of informative and invaluable literature and various aids which they offer to dentists, to schools and to clinics, and the dental profession should be grateful to them for this. The public is now very much better informed as a result, and has become so at a very much earlier age – vital in terms of effective prevention. Dental practitioners, too, ought to take a lot of the credit, for many are now much more involved in prevention in terms of hygiene and diet. If all could become so – and it is basically only an outdated NHS remuneration system that holds many dentists back – then dentists could save the country millions and millions of pounds. If dentists could be enabled to become health and hygiene consultants rather than dreaded drillers, the dental health of the British could improve enormously and the cost of living in Britain could reduce in proportion.

Sugar and Tooth Decay

As saliva plus bacteria equals plaque, so it can be said that plaque plus sugar equals acid equals tooth decay. But, of course, as in anything, it's not quite that simple. All of us can probably point to an individual who eats sweets all day, never brushes his teeth, never goes to the dentist, and who never seems to develop any tooth decay; and all of us know of people who are dentally very conscientious, and yet who suffer endlessly from decay problems. Sadly, it is an indisputable fact that some people are just more vulnerable to decay than others. This could be hereditary or genetic, but it's primarily a matter of individual biochemistry: it could be that the enamel did not calcify properly, it could be that the major acid-producing bacteria are very much more prolific in a particular mouth; or it could be that the body is just rather acidic in nature. The breakdown of the biochemistry in an individual mouth can be likened to those dominos which are made to fall down in progression: even if only one of the mouth factors already mentioned alters or is altered in some way – the oral bacteria, the shape of the teeth, the content and flow of the saliva, the way in which the mouth is used – then that delicate inter-reaction is altered as well, the dominos start to fall, and disease or tooth decay could be the result.

But sugar, of course, despite individual variances in vulnerability and resistance, is still the principal cause of tooth decay, and it is its interaction with plaque in the mouth that starts the process off. This fairly modern theory of caries or tooth decay is attributed to one W. B. Millar. At the end of the last century he incubated teeth with saliva and carbohydrates; acid was formed and some of the calcium on the teeth was dissolved. When no carbohydrate was incubated, no dissolving took place, so he concluded that carbohydrate was needed to cause tooth decay.

THE SUGAR THAT WE EAT

Sugar is a carbohydrate along with the starches, and starch carbohydrates are valuable to the body in that they are a useful and often cheap source of energy. The unrefined complex carbohydrates found in vegetables, fruit, pulses and whole grains are the best type you can eat, as they provide vitamins, minerals and trace elements as well as dietary fibre. Most carbohydrates in a western diet, however, have been so refined and concentrated that they are virtually empty foods, stripped of any nutritional value. The most empty carbohydrate of all is processed sugar, for it provides only calories and nothing else whatsoever, and is actually *put into* a vast number of foods. Sugar could truthfully be described as one of the major evils of civilization for it is dangerous in so many ways apart from its undoubted dental effect: it can be directly linked with a multitude of other bodily ills. In fact, as one well-known expert has said, sugar is known to be so dangerous that if it began to be marketed as a drug, it would be immediately banned.

All the sugars that we eat are potentially harmful dentally, but the most dangerous are the most refined, the most sticky and the most powdered. Even the natural sugars found in fruit and vegetables (fructose) and milk (lactose) *could*, if conditions in the mouth were bad enough, lead to acid production, for virtually any carbohydrate – even the non-sugar starches – can eventually, if given long enough, produce acid which then produces tooth decay. Other sugars which are considered more natural are honey and the unrefined cane sugars, and they do undoubtedly contain many good things nutritionally: dentally, however, they are just as damaging, honey particularly as it is so viscous and sticky.

And the more refined a sugar, the more empty, the more dead, and the more dangerous it becomes. The gleaming white crystalline table sugar that is sprinkled on cereals or stirred into hot drinks, and the icing sugar that makes Christmas cake frostings, are the worst of all. If you consider that the average amount of sugar eaten per week by every man, woman and child in the UK is 900 g (2 lb), then it can come as no surprise that we are still a country ravaged by the horrors of tooth decay. Now that many more people are aware of the dangers of sugar to teeth and weight, some have changed to a low sugar diet – and this means, as the figures have remained unchanged, that some others are eating more, at least their weight again in sugar per year!

For, although the consumption of white sugar has dropped, the consumption of confectionery has increased; sugar may have been dropped from tea or coffee, but a sweet craving – for sugar *is* addictive – still continues, and is being satisfied by confectionery. About 110 g (4 oz) of that average 900 g (2 lb) sugar is consumed in the form of confectionery. Children consume twice the national average of sweets thus can consume up to 225 g (8 oz) of sugar per week – some children can eat up to 225 g (8 oz) of sugar *per day*. As children are especially vulnerable to tooth decay, what with mass advertising and mass availability of sweet things, they can take too much and become victims to obesity and early diabetes as well.

It's a social conditioning to believe that sweets are a 'treat'; a more truthful statement would be that sweets are a 'poison', and any product which contains a large percentage of sugar – 10 per cent, say – should carry the message: DANGER: HEALTH WARNING. THIS PRODUCT CONTAINS SUGAR WHICH CAN SERIOUSLY DAMAGE YOUR HEALTH, just as on cigarette packets. We could also tax sweets – for they are basically a non-nutritious food – and profits could go towards anti-sugar advertising. Perhaps the day might come when sugar and sweet manufacturers could be *sued* for the amount of pain and suffering their wares cause: drug manufacturers are sued, after all, and a cigarette company in the States has recently been sued by the family of someone who died from lung cancer. The sweet manufacturers are less than reasonably responsible about their role in tooth decay. They have even tried to persuade us that the oils or fats in some sweets can *prevent* decay. It is true that nut and seed oils are thought to inhibit the bacteria lying on the teeth, but the oils of chocolate surely could not hope to counteract the amount of sugar in it – up to 65 per cent in some chocolate caramel bars!

But it is not just sweets that contain refined sugar. A staggering number of other products do as well – and they are the hidden sugars. Cakes, sweetened cereals, biscuits, jams, fruits canned in syrup, even dried fruit, and chocolate drinks are obvious, but less obvious are 'health' cereals, bread, things like canned tomato soup – which contains 10 per cent sucrose – tomato ketchup, canned peas, beans and spaghetti, and corned beef! Get into the habit of reading the contents labels of refined foods – packets, bags and cans etc. – and the number of unlikely things that contain sugar will amaze you. Remember that, like baby foods, the ingredients are listed in descending order of quantity: sugar near the head of the list means a large proportion of sugar. In fact labelling, which is happily becoming more common, ought to list the *type* of sugar as well, and the percentage of sugar that is present. We could then easily avoid them. For, although many supermarket chains are becoming more aware of the public dislike for sugar and other additives, the only way to truly convince all manufacturers is simply not to buy their goods until they are forced to take sugar out of their products.

There is sugar in many medicines as well – in antibiotics, laxatives, cough syrups, vitamins, tranquillizers and anti-depressants – and it is particularly horrifying that liquid baby medicines are high in sucrose. Manufacturers like to use sugar syrup as a base because it is cheap, the flavour masks the principal active ingredients, and it helps the medicine to have a longer shelf life. There is obviously an assumption too that babies will more readily *take* a medicine with a sweet taste, and doctors and dentists should be fighting vigorously against this. There *are* now some baby medicines which are sugar-free, but of the antibiotics, say – probably the most commonly prescribed in infancy and childhood — there are, from one survey, twenty-one *with* sugar and only one without.

WHEN SUGAR IS MOST DAMAGING

A high-sugar diet is one in which sugar is taken at frequent intervals, even if it is in small amounts. And it is the *frequency* of sugar consumption that is the most damaging in both body and dental terms. One cream cake a week for a treat (although I dislike that word and concept), or in an unavoidable social circumstance, probably won't do a great deal of harm. But it's the snack foods eaten between meals when saliva production is low, and the sugar taken in those frequent cups of tea or coffee throughout the day that is likely to produce the most acid, and thus the potential for the most tooth decay. For each time sugar comes in touch with plaque, the acid produced will stay on the teeth for up to twenty minutes. The sugar will not *clear* from the teeth for that time, and the chart shows the acidogenicity of some common foods. It's like stoking a boiler: the more sugar that is put in, the more acid will be produced, and the production of acid will go on for longer.

Acidogenicity of common snack foods

Most acidogenic		
	1	Boiled sweet (fruit-flavoured)
	2	Sugared coffee
	3	Toffee
	4	Orange drink (sweetened)
	5	Plain biscuit (sweet)
	6	Sugared chewing gum
	7	Chocolate biscuit
	8	Sweet chocolate
	9	Ice cream
	10	Cream-filled biscuit
	11	Apple
	12	Chocolate/caramel bar
	13	Chocolate-covered peanuts
	14	Cough syrup
	15	Unsugared coffee
	16	Ice lolly (frozen fruit drink)
	17	Potato crisps
	18	Bread and butter
	19	Peanuts
Least acidogenic	20	Sugar-free chewing gum

Adapted from the work of W. M. Edgar, reproduced in *Diet, Nutrition and Dentistry* by Randolph and Dennison (The C. V. Mosby Company, 1981)

Smokers who suck minty sweets regularly to sweeten their breaths (and sucking is worse than chewing), are very prone to this prolonged acid attack – and when they give up smoking it can be even worse in their new need for an alternate oral stimulation! If a mint is sucked every ten minutes, throughout the day, the effects in terms of acid production will be worse than if *ten packets* of mints were consumed all in one go. Similarly, it's no good people claiming that they only have 1 teaspoon of sugar in each drink if they actually have ten cups of coffee per day: they would be better having one cup containing 10 teaspoons of sugar!

The consistency of sugar is also a major danger, and the classic dentist's horror is the chocolate-coated, soft caramel bar which is full of sucrose and is sticky. The fineness of the sucrose will lower the pH of the mouth much more drastically because it dissolves so quickly (which is why fizzy drinks are so bad: the sucrose is already dissolved). The stickiness of the sucrose will contribute similarly to a rapid lowering of the pH and will also stick to the plaque on the tooth for longer; the saliva will not be able to wash it away easily.

Although sugar is undeniably bad for teeth and for health in general, there is another aspect of sugar consumption which is extremely worrying. All the carbohydrates supply energy, and most of them do so more cheaply and nutritiously than sugar. But many sugar-eating children are gaining their energy solely from their sugar-coated cereals, sweets and ice creams, and thus are not eating the good foods. The classic example is of the child who does not have room for proper meals but who is satisfying hunger and energy needs through snack foods. If that child had not developed a sweet tooth, had not been allowed to eat sugary foods, and those sugary foods had simply not been available, he would have been able to satisfy himself on the more complex carbohydrates which would satisfy him *for longer*, and to a far higher nutritional standard. Many children who constantly eat sweet and refined things can be technically as severely malnourished as children who have no food at all.

SUGAR AND CHILDREN'S TEETH

Tooth decay on baby teeth can be an unmitigated disaster, as already described. This really must be one of the worst ways in which sugar can work its dreadful effects and thus sugar should be avoided at all costs. Decay can be caused by dummies dipped in honey which are constantly in the mouth, therefore constantly creating acid – for baby teeth have plaque just as do permanent teeth. Other villains are the sweet syrupy drinks for children, perhaps left in a feeding bottle for the baby or child to suck.

A very small amount of tooth decay on a baby tooth can cause damage quite out of proportion to the amount of decay: because teeth are so small, the smallest cavity can damage the nerve or cause an abscess. Once the cavity is established, because the structure of the deciduous enamel is thinner and weaker, the tooth can tend to break. Teeth which decay at an early age might need filling more than once or even twice by the time they are eventually shed, and the psychological effects of these treatments on a young four- or five-year-old can be very distressing indeed. Avoidance of sugar during the period of deciduous dentition is vital, as the teeth are really not designed to go bad.

Tooth decay can also seriously affect the first permanent teeth to erupt – usually the first molars which come in at about six years. The tooth is more porous at this stage and much more chemically active, so that lots of good and bad chemicals can get into the surface enamel. Sugar at this rather vocal stage – the classic time when children start to demand sweets (coinciding with going to school, perhaps?) – can be disastrous as holes can appear virtually overnight because of this increased enamel permeability. This is when, as already noted, topical fluoride should be applied, as a lot of it will soak into the tooth's surface. It's rather like painting a rough unseasoned piece of wood, when the first coat literally soaks into the grain.

The avoidance of sugar is still the greatest priority though, for sugar control is more important in preventing tooth decay than any other measure, and this is perhaps the *only* thing on which all dentists agree! As a profession we have been lobbying for years, but against the bureaucratic and financial might of the opposing lobby – the sugar and sweet manufacturers, to whom the yearly UK consumption of sugar is worth 300 million pounds – our voices echo in the wilderness. As a result our main effort has been diverted into looking at cheaper and more effective ways of preventing tooth decay – and thus the concentration on fluoride.

It's a fudging of the issue really, and a treating of the effects, not the cause: the principal thrust of prevention ought still to be to eliminate refined sugar entirely from everyone's diet.

The Progression of Tooth Decay

From pelicule to plaque formation, then from sugar intake to acid production to dissolved calcium is a chronological chemical process which could be compared to the rusting on a car. Water on the metal produces a chemical which then oxidizes or dissolves the surface of the metal; the rusting may only reveal itself at first as a few small bubbles on the paint surface, but once the paint is stripped away, there could be a massive amount of rust and destruction beneath. Similarly, decay on a tooth which may look minimal on the surface enamel could have spread underneath the enamel, throughout the dentine, to create a much more destructive cavity.

THE EARLY STAGES AND REMINERALIZATION

Early tooth decay is in essence a *de*mineralization of the tooth's surface. The acid dissolves the minerals out of the enamel, and the plaque, which has the capacity to soak up vast amounts of calcium, draws the minerals into itself. At this early stage, visible signs might be little white spots on the enamel – the zones of attack from acid; the decay might not be felt at all, or the tooth might react to hot or cold, especially the latter. This is the time when the two-way process, the ebb and flow of minerals, can affect the tooth decay and its progression. Once this early tooth decay is present, it does not mean that it necessarily has to get worse. If the body and mouth environments change or are adjusted correctly – through a good diet primarily – the saliva can deposit more minerals to replace those taken out. Through a good diet and the use of topical fluoride, these spots of early tooth decay can be slowed up or stopped; there is every likelihood that the tooth can regenerate, that the tooth can repair itself.

CAVITIES

Once the acid breaches the calcium and reaches the dentine, however, cavities are created, when the bacteria can wreak their toxic havoc, and dental fillings will probably be necessary. This is what could formally be called the end of possible remineralization, and is the time when the dentist has to clinically make up his mind what the next step might be. If there is a *very small* cavity, it could remain static if good diet and meticulous hygiene were followed: it could be left and merely checked every year or so by X-ray, to see if it had grown any bigger. Again this is a decision a dentist has to make, weighing up the general body and mouth health of the patient in order to assess a possible *rate* of tooth decay progression.

Once a cavity has been created that is big enough for the bacteria to live in, they can begin to have a toxic effect themselves; it is no longer just the acid they produce that is damaging. They are in a sheltered haven, out of reach of toothbrush, floss and toothpaste; there is plenty of fermentable carbohydrate constantly reaching into the cavity; and upon this and the tooth itself they can feed at leisure and without fear of attack; and, although the saliva *can* reach in, it has to do so through a jungle of bacteria and the buffering effect will therefore not be so great. The more the 'cave' effect of the cavity, the more the bacteria have free rein, and the greater the likelihood that a filling will have to be inserted.

The most likely parts of the tooth to decay are the areas which are difficult to clean thoroughly. These are the fissures on the biting surfaces of the molars, in between tight teeth or merely teeth that touch each other, and the border between teeth and gums. So tooth decay can occur on the top of teeth, at the sides, or in between teeth, and in all cases the acids can eat through to the dentine. If undetected and left unfilled, the bacteria will spread rapidly through the dentine, and pass along its tiny canals to infect the pulp at the heart of the tooth. An increased blood supply bringing extra white cells to fight the infection will inflame the pulp. This presses on the nerves and will cause toothache. However, if detected early by the dentist, the decay can be removed, and the cavity shaped; a calcium lining placed over the nerve area and then a filling material can be inserted, and both pain and decay will have been arrested.

It is the saliva which is influential to a great extent in determining which areas of the mouth tend to have tooth decay and which don't, but often you can have an even more extraordinary situation. This is where, on a single tooth, one part is developing tooth decay while another part has a deposition of tartar: two completely different chemical processes within millimetres of each other. This shows the complexity of the situation, and there are many theories concerning calcium and phosphate concentrations. Another circumstance is when two teeth are adjacent and therefore could reasonably be expected to share the same bacteria and the same plaque. One tooth can have a large decay cavity while the one next door will show no signs of decay at all. The biochemistry of the mouth, of the formation of the teeth, and of the process and progression of tooth decay is *very* subtle, and only requires the most minor change for it to swing out of balance.

ABSCESSES

An abscess occurs when the bacteria and the putrefying products of the cavity – in nerve or pulp – pour out of the end of the tooth into the bone. Pus gathers and inflammation spreads, often accompanied by a facial colouring and swelling. Although tooth decay isn't life-threatening, dental abscesses derived from tooth decay *can* be if allowed to spread and if not controlled by, say, the use of antibiotics. In the upper jaw, the mode of drainage of infected tissue is often upwards and it can run perilously close to the brain tissue: infected material which does drain upwards can join vessels that run into the brain to cause brain infection and possible death. Similarly, in the lower jaw, the swelling in the neck following a dental abscess could be so severe that it obstructs the breathing and causes death through asphyxiation.

This, however, is unlikely in 'civilized' western society where dentists and doctors are easily available to relieve pain and to control infection – but the potential is there if totally neglected, and certainly was a cause of death before the advent of antibiotics. And, indeed, although holistic practitioners do not believe in the use of drugs unless absolutely necessary, antibiotics may be of the essence when attempting to control a dental abscess. In many cases a dentist can see and lance an abscess if it's on the surface, allowing the pus to drain out into the mouth; often, however, the

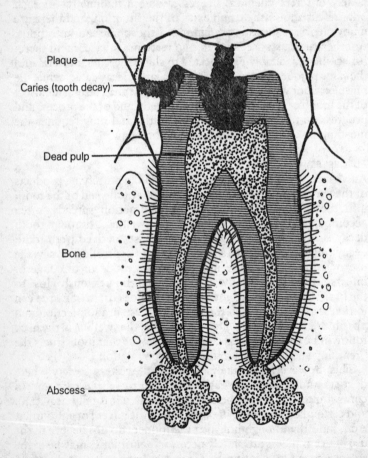

Plaque

Caries (tooth decay)

Dead pulp

Bone

Abscess

Tooth decay and abscess

pus will burrow its way inwards through the bone so that the dentist cannot see it or treat it other than by antibiotics.

RAMPANT TOOTH DECAY

The difference between rampant tooth decay and tooth decay as we would normally see it is that the former occurs all over the mouth and at greater speed. Dentists know where to look for the beginnings of tooth-decay cavities – some areas in the average person's dentition are more likely to be affected. But rampant tooth decay can cover virtually every tooth, and every surface can be affected.

In rampant tooth decay there is little ebb and flow of reminer-alization: it's all a one-way process. The whole tooth is destroyed at a very much more rapid rate: the bacteria inside the tooth multiply phenomenally quickly, and physically eat away the interior and surface of the tooth. The nerve can be exposed very quickly because it hasn't got time to lay down the protective secondary dentine, and large chunks of the tooth can break off under pressure.

The actual colour and texture of rampant tooth decay are different from the more slowly developing ordinary tooth decay. The texture is often soft and cheese-like, and is also much lighter in colour. In ordinary tooth decay, a dentist would have to use a fairly slow drill to scrape the decay away in layers; in rampant tooth decay, he can literally *scoop* the decay out of the tooth. Rampant tooth decay often shows itself as a tiny hole on the surface, and because of its light coloration, it is often not noticed; underneath, however, the whole tooth is a mush. Rampant tooth decay is both distressing because it is very painful, and disfiguring because it occurs on all parts of the mouth, even affecting teeth which are normally very much less prone to tooth decay.

Rampant tooth decay is generally related to age and to diet. Individuals who suffer from it can often be juveniles in their teens who have social problems, and who have poor nutrition and bad salivary flow as a result. They can be psychologically disadvan-taged as well, with repressed emotions, feelings of inferiority and rebellion, and can be pasty in complexion, and slow learners. This is not dependent on heredity, but entirely on diet, when the body just cannot cope with the poor nutrition. It is also interesting to relate these facts to the recent findings about the relationship between poor diet, mood and personality, and levels of juvenile delinquency. Boys in Borstals have been shown to change personality when given a good diet after years, possibly, on a poor one. I expect many of them could have been suffering from rampant tooth decay as well.

However, bad hygiene can also produce rampant tooth decay, as can a diminution of salivary fluid due to disease. There is a decay process which could almost be called rampant, too, and this occurs in older people who develop a mild form of diabetes, giving them a constant hankering for sweet things. Although their teeth are older and therefore should be more chemically mature and resistant, there is often a lot of root recession, and decay can start there. This root decay progresses very quickly, often at a similar rate to rampant tooth decay, and can result in teeth snapping off.

CAN TOOTH DECAY BE CONTAGIOUS?

In the sense of normal infection, one person cannot, of course, infect another with tooth decay. But there are three ways in which tooth decay may be said to be transmitted. The first is the genetic factor already discussed, in that it can happen that children inherit a poorer tooth structure or a crowded jaw, and thus a greater vulnerability to tooth decay, from their parents. The second is the acquisition of the wrong bacteria, the image of a hypothetical midwife who might transmit 'tooth decay bacteria' to a new baby. Bacteria can be transmitted from mouth to mouth on the breath, or by kissing, say, but it's not a true form of contagion, in that most adult mouths will possess the whole range of the same bacteria anyway. Even if new bacteria were introduced to one mouth, the potential development of tooth decay depends on how that body, mouth and saliva modify them: new acquired bacteria do not necessarily mean a transmitted disease. Even kissing someone who has rampant tooth decay does not mean that the other will develop rampant tooth decay too: but it might be a better idea to point out the unacceptability of rampant tooth decay, and refuse to kiss until the sufferer had his teeth seen and treated by a dentist!

The final and major way in which I think one could say that tooth decay is transmittable is through parents feeding their children a bad diet. Parents who allow unlimited access to the classic tooth-decay foods – sweets, biscuits, cakes, fizzy drinks – are in effect infecting their children: they could truly be said to be transmitting disease to their children.

Tooth Decay and Pain

The relationship between tooth decay and pain, surprisingly, is not clear. Dentists often see people with teeth decayed to the gumline, teeth reduced to black stumps, teeth with nerves exposed, teeth with abscesses – but when they ask how severe the discomfort is, the answer often is that the 'sufferer' hasn't known a day's pain in his life! And conversely, a patient can have the tiniest early decay mark in a tooth, and can feel quite a lot of discomfort. The perception of pain varies enormously from patient to patient – it must be one of the most difficult and variable sensations to describe and to judge – but it does bear a direct relationship to stress. If someone is under severe stress, it is well known that their pain threshold – the point at which they actually perceive pain – is lowered so that even the smallest stimulus can cause pain. This sounds as if it might be psychological, but in fact it is very physical: biochemical tests have shown that nerve reactions are actually at a higher pitch, and when someone claims that their 'nerves are on edge', it's not too far removed from a basic biological truth.

If pain occurs in a tooth, it doesn't necessarily mean the tooth has a hole in it: there are a number of other causes, and even a mild coronary could give the sensation of toothache. A reaction to hot and cold, say, can be due to the dentine being exposed on a tooth. The symptoms can be the same as early tooth decay, and the solution may be just to use a palliative toothpaste, or the dentist can seal over the areas with a desensitizing liquid. This sensitivity can be caused by over-enthusiastic toothbrushing or gum recession, but it can also be brought on by stress. If pain is generalized – in more than one part of the mouth – the dentist would be more justified in looking into the cause of the stress, rather than treating the effects.

The classic toothache situation begins, though, when a tooth-decay cavity extends into the dentine and bacteria are irritating the tissues. This could cause the early reactions to hot and cold or a minor occasional discomfort. If this is allowed to continue, it will often deteriorate into a pain of longer duration. This is when the decay has spread and toxins and even bacteria may be entering the nerve of the tooth. This is followed by a very severe constant pain which can be excruciating, and has been described by many as the very worst pain that can be perceived. This is often associated with the nerve dying, and once that happens, the severe pain may suddenly cease, to be succeeded by a painless state, or simply a dull sensation. Within a day or two, however, the follow-up could be the characteristic pain of an abscess.

Even when the tooth is treated early, dentists cannot guarantee that their treatment will miraculously cause the cessation of pain. The tooth and its layers form a biological structure which will take time to heal, and the treatment itself – the drilling, vibration, the cold air, the heat generated by the drill – can also upset the delicate nerve structure. Thus, after a filling, there is often a continuing sense of discomfort, but as the process of healing progresses, this should diminish.

Obviously the first priority of the dentist is to relieve the pain being experienced by the patient. To gauge the type of pain and attempt to locate the trouble, he will have to ask a barrage of questions. When does the pain occur? What is the stimulus? As pain thresholds of individual patients can vary so much, this can be a difficult exercise unless there is a fairly accurate response. Soon, however, the dentist should be able to discover the cause of the pain and the severity of damage to the nerve, and his treatment will be appropriate to that. The problem can be very complex, though, for with a molar, say, which has three roots, there could be one root dead, one half dead, and one alive: and these could show each and every pain symptom from reaction to hot and cold on one root to a full-blown abscess on the other with its accompanying pain and tenderness. Diagnosis isn't easy.

The one-time first option of dentists was to remove a tooth that was causing pain. Nowadays, with the advent of various treatments like root canal therapy, teeth can be saved even if they have been allowed to decay and abscess. Apart from teeth suffering from rampant tooth decay, there aren't many teeth that cannot be saved by modern dentistry, given that their structure and their position in the bone are solid.

The Prevention of Tooth Decay

Just as even the most minor alteration in one of the chemical factors in the mouth can cause tooth decay, so the knocking out of one or more of the factors which *contribute* to tooth decay can make the decay rate decrease dramatically or indeed cease completely. If hygiene is improved, tooth decay can be lessened; if sugar is omitted from the diet, teeth will be far healthier; if attendance at the dentist is regular, incipient tooth decay can be spotted and treated. These basic principles have been reiterated almost ad nauseam, but they are still major factors in prevention. Science, too, has been investigating ways of preventing tooth decay: an anti-decay vaccine has been under investigation for at least forty years; research has suggested that antibiotics can cause a reduction of the bacterial content in the mouth; and a lot of the toothpaste manufacturers have been working on enzymes which would inhibit the conversion of carbohydrates into acid. Topical fluoride, too, has an important role in the prevention of tooth decay, and I discuss that in the next chapter. However, from personal experience, from population study researches, and from the work of many experts throughout the world, the one overriding factor in low or non-existent tooth decay appears to be diet. It's the one factor which I feel is relevant and which is consistent.

The first principles involve many of the elements discussed in earlier chapters, and relate to the earliest possible prevention. The good spacing of teeth within a well-shaped jaw will mean less decay. This can be achieved by good diet during pregnancy and infancy. The shape of a tooth can be a factor in tooth decay, for if it has awkward cusps and lots of fissures, bacteria and food debris can more easily remain on the tooth. Although I believe the morphology or shape of the teeth is dependent on a number of factors, including that of genetics, there is a strong argument that deep fissures in teeth are caused by nutritional deficiencies during calcification. The chemical structure of the tooth, too, is indubitably connected with nutrition, in that the minerals and trace elements so vital for good mineralization of the teeth can easily be ingested from good diet, again during pregnancy and infancy.

Good spacing of teeth, even teeth and chemically sound teeth, then, are significant factors in the fight against tooth decay, and they are the result of good nutrition. The chemistry of the mouth too is vital, for the saliva is all important. If the saliva could be rich enough in its preventative factors, it could reduce the bacterial count and inhibit their reproduction. If the saliva has a good flow and viscosity rate, there is less tooth decay; there is more washing-away and buffering effect, and fresh enzymes are being produced. Saliva is intimately connected with health of the body in general, and health of the body is dependent on diet.

The avoidance of sugar is an obvious dietary necessity, and a good wholefood diet must be followed. And by eating the tough fibrous foods of a good diet – raw fruit, raw vegetables, whole grains etc. – not only the health of body will be improved, but the teeth could be cleaned as well. Chewing and chomping could actually have a detergent effect and help the saliva to dislodge and wash away much of the bacteria and plaque. The hard bite of many who eat foods that are crunchy can also be a factor: minerals from the food can be ground into the surface of the tooth, to form a harder, less permeable layer. The pressure and banging can harden up the layers underneath as well, so that the dentine appears thicker and stronger. Heavy mastication, then, can help prevent tooth decay, as can the chewing effect itself of course – for that, in its turn, produces more saliva. It's all swings and roundabouts. However, the crunchy apple a day that is commonly thought to keep the doctor and dentist away (or at bay?) could be less of a friend: apples are acidic thus produce a low pH in the mouth, and if they're eaten after sugars – as they so often are, for their supposedly magical washing-away effect – they can actually make the situation worse! Although foods can be detergent, brushing and flossing should remain the principal means of cleaning.

I have talked about acidity and alkalinity levels in the mouth – the pH scale – but this could indeed be even more closely linked with the body and diet. For the body too has an ideal acid/alkaline balance, and the foods that the body ingests – which are either acid- or alkaline-forming – can affect this balance. If too many acid-forming foods – coffee, sugar, meat and processed foods in general – are eaten, they can cause an extremely acid response in the body. This contributes directly to many illnesses such as arthritis – indeed stress itself produces an acid response in the body – but if the saliva and oral juices are influenced by the body generally, this acid body reaction could form an even more acidic saliva. If we could produce alkaline reactions in the body through alkaline-forming foods such as fresh raw fruit and vegetables, we might be able to produce an alkaline saliva which could combat any acidic effects very much more effectively. This is pure speculation, but it could be a further – and very significant – dietary way of preventing tooth decay.

To sum up in general, it must always be remembered that tooth decay is an entirely preventable disease. Provided there is regular attendance at the dentist, a good diet is followed, and oral hygiene is effective, no one should ever need to have too much dental treatment or lose a tooth through decay. However, given all that, you might take a horse to water, but you can't make it drink. Unfortunately, there seems to be a resistance to advice, and thus we still have dental disease. It's *not* because there's a lack of information, it's the lack of putting that information into practice. Tooth decay, therefore, is very relevant still and, unless there's a complete change of heart from all (unlikely, I fear), it will remain so into the foreseeable future.

CHAPTER SIX

Fluoride

It is ironic that the relationship fluoride has with our teeth was not discovered through its beneficial effects, but because it causes unsightly stains and mottling. This was over fifty years ago, and since then there have been arguments for and against using fluoride to help prevent tooth decay. At the level of one part per million (fluoride to water), there appears to be very little evidence to suggest that fluoride has any side effects. This is the recommended concentration, and it has been shown to effectively protect the tooth from tooth decay. However, it must be remembered that fluoride is potentially a very toxic element and it is already present in our food, beverages, drugs, aerosols, non-stick pans, and fibreglass, as well as in fluoride tablets and toothpaste. We are surrounded, in a sense, by fluoride, and the real debate as I see it is how we can control and monitor a 'safe' level in our bodies.

Fluorine

Fluorine is a very active element chemically and is similar in many ways to chlorine. Both are very poisonous and readily combine with metals to form stable salts. Chlorine will combine with sodium to form sodium chloride, or common salt. Fluorine will behave in a similar way, giving a white sodium fluoride which also tastes salty. When fluoride reacts with other materials the resulting compound is often chemically stable. This reaction benefits our teeth by preventing them dissolving in the acids produced in the dental plaque. But many are worried that this 'stabilizing' influence may, if fluoride is present in our bodies in large amounts, have an *adverse* effect, locking up the vital minerals and enzymes necessary for good biological function.

DOSAGE AND THE EFFECTS ON TEETH

The deciduous or 'baby' teeth do not appear to be substantially affected by fluoride during their formation. The evidence indicates that little or no fluoride passes through the placental membrane, and thus, for those who wish to take fluoride supplements during pregnancy, there appears to be little advantage. But the permanent teeth are affected by fluoride and the dosage appears to be an all-important factor. Concentrations of up to one part per million (1 ppm) appear to have few or no side effects on the enamel of the teeth. In fact, many have observed that the enamel appears more pearly white and uniform in structure, so it would seem that the fluoride not only makes the teeth more resistant to decay, but also makes them 'harder' and cosmetically more pleasing.

There appears to be little leeway before mottling is evident on the teeth. Many authorities agree that 1.5 ppm is the approximate concentration when signs of fluorosis may occur, and at 2 ppm, up to 10 per cent of the teeth could show areas of brown stains or dull white opaque patches. At 4 ppm as few as one or two teeth only are *not* affected, with many badly stained and blotchy. Some of the teeth may also have pitting of the surface enamel, and where there are brown stains, the enamel may be structurally weaker. The effects of fluorosis can penetrate the complete thickness of the enamel, so intense brushing is unlikely to alter the colour or staining of the damaged teeth.

Let's look at the dosage in perspective. One part per million means adding the equivalent of one tiny grain of salt to a cup of water. This can be described as a beneficial dose. What is of concern to me is that 2 grains can have a harmful effect! We are all individuals and no more so than in our dietary habits. Can we standardize how much water we consume, how much tea we drink, or how much fish we eat? – for both tea and fish skin contain quite significant amounts of fluoride. If we are given a standard dose of any substance do we react in a standardized way? The answer is no.

FLUORIDE AND TOOTH DECAY

The popular impression is that fluoride protects the tooth by giving the enamel a protective invisible shield. This is partly true as the enamel is made more resistant to attack from acids just as paint will help to protect a car from rusting. The fluoride does appear to concentrate on the surface of the enamel thereby forming a less soluble layer. Fluoride will also influence the activity of the bacteria in the plaque. It does this in two ways: by interfering with the growth and behaviour of the bacteria close to the surface of the tooth, and by modifying the biochemical reactions which actually produce the acid. Both of these demonstrate how fluoride is a powerful enzyme inhibitor. Fluoride also acts like a chemical 'buffer', reducing the activity of the acids and in effect neutralizing them. Another beneficial reaction to which fluoride contributes on the surface of the tooth is to encourage the saliva to 'heal' the enamel by laying down new minerals.

It has been observed that when fluoride has been taken during the formation of the teeth, their shape may be slightly altered. The molars may have wider and shallower fissures. This has the obvious advantages of reducing potential hiding places for bacteria and facilitating cleaning. Fluoride concentration in the teeth increases with age and this may be one of the reasons why the rate of tooth decay will often reduce as one becomes older.

Systemic Fluorides

Systemic means the inclusion of a substance into the whole body, and therefore systemic fluorides are those which, besides being incorporated into the tooth, can also be metabolized and included into all the body tissues.

FLUORIDATION OF WATER SUPPLIES

After many years of debate, Parliament in Britain has passed a bill enabling the health authorities to introduce fluoride into water supplies. Due to financial and technical difficulties, this does not mean that all areas of the country are fluoridated at the moment, but it does give the legal means whereby this can be achieved. Fluoridation has been introduced as a form of mass medication for the sole purpose of helping to prevent tooth decay. I believe it is a sad day when a nation has to be medicated because of a general failing in its diet and oral hygiene habits. And there is, of course, an ethical consideration – that of the right to choose.

Many have fears that it is virtually impossible to control the total fluoride doses our bodies may receive, and this is magnified by the inclusion of fluoride in our drinking water. Babies drink large amounts of fluid compared to their body weight and should their nutrients be mixed and diluted with fluoridated water, this would be in addition to the existing concentration of fluoride already present in their food. If these foods have been produced or grown in an area of fluoridation, there must be concern about the amount of fluoride these tiny bodies are ingesting.

When food is processed using fluoridated water, the concentration of fluoride can increase dramatically: Gouda cheese, for instance, normally contains 27 mg per kg of fluoride, but after processing with fluoridated water at 1 ppm, the levels of fluoride in the cheese can be increased by a factor of 10. Fruit and vegetables may also concentrate fluoride if there is an abundance in the soil. In fluoridated areas the watering of plants would be a source of this increase. Fluoride is also contained in some fertilizers and pesticides. Tea contains fluoride, and many people can drink five or more cups a day. Reports of twenty cups a day are not uncommon. If the water to make the tea also contains fluoride the daily intake may well exceed recommended safety levels.

The main disadvantage appears to be that by indiscriminately adding fluoride to the water there can be no control on a chemical whose effect on the body we do not fully comprehend. The counter claim is that fluoridation of our drinking water is a cost-effective way of considerably reducing the level of tooth decay in the population: figures of over 50 per cent reduction in decay have been quoted from comparative surveys, and would be of benefit to those members of our society whose priority does not lie in the care of their teeth.

FLUORIDE TABLETS AND DROPS

At present a large majority of dentists recommend fluoride drops or tablets as a method of systemic fluoridation if their patients live in an area where the level of fluoride in the water supply is low.

Because of the increasing concern about the risk of mottling of teeth dentists will normally follow a dosage regime similar to the table set out below:

Recommended fluoride supplementation (in mg fluoride ion) (Foman and Wei 1976)

Fluoride concentration of water supply	AGE 0–6 months	AGE 6–18 months	AGE 18–36 months	AGE 3–6 yrs.	AGE > 6 yrs.
< 0.2	0	0.25	0.5	0.75	1.00
0.2–0.4	0	0	0.25	0.50	0.75
0.4–0.6	0	0	0	0.25	0.50
0.6–0.8	0	0	0	0	0.25
> 0.8	0	0	0	0	0

From *Current Aspects of Dental Health*, Cooper Products, 1983

If you do want to start young children on fluoride drops or tablets, seek professional advice from a dentist. In the USA many medical doctors are now taking the responsibility for the supervision of fluoride administration. If the child is old enough, fluoride tablets are better sucked or chewed so that the fluoride can have an additional topical effect. There do seem to be considerable benefits as regards the reduction of tooth decay by the use of fluoride drops and tablets, but a disadvantage is that of maintaining a continuous daily intake throughout the period of tooth formation and eruption. It is also very important to keep fluoride tablets locked in the medicine cupboard as an overdose can be very serious. If such an unfortunate eventuality occurs then you should obtain medical advice and treatment as soon as possible, induce vomiting, and give milk antacids or lime water to drink.

The question, 'Should I give my children fluoride tablets?' is one I find difficult to answer. Fluoride *will* help protect the teeth, but I believe in the philosophy when prescribing drugs, that 'if in doubt – don't'. I am not convinced that enough research has been undertaken into the effects fluoride may have on our bones, organs, enzyme systems and essential mineral reserves.

Both pro- and anti-fluoridation camps present statistics to

enforce their arguments, but we all know how statistics can be presented to cast beneficial light on one's own point of view. Lack of fluoride is not the cause of tooth decay – poor diet and poor oral hygiene is. It is ironic that the parents of children who are conscientious enough to enquire about fluoride administration are also the same parents who will ensure good supervision of home dental care and make sure their children have a low refined carbohydrate intake. Just the sort of parents whose children would most probably *not* require systemic fluoride! Fluoride *is* undeniably beneficial to our teeth so why don't we concentrate on enriching the surface layers of the enamel rather than the whole body.

Topical Fluorides

This describes any method of fluoridation when the fluoride is applied directly on to the tooth.

FLUORIDE TOOTHPASTES

One of the best methods of applying fluoride to the teeth is by using toothpaste. Nearly all (over 90 per cent) of dentifrices sold in the UK contain a fluoride supplement. I am sure that fluoride toothpaste has played a significant role in the present reduction in the amount of tooth decay. Different manufacturers use different systems to 'deliver' fluoride on to the surface enamel, and the concentration of fluoride in toothpaste can be as high as 1500 parts per million. Thus it is very important to supervise children when they are brushing their teeth, if only to ensure that they do not swallow or eat the paste. Disturbing stories of children making 'toothpaste butties' and spearmint toothpaste drinks must be a warning to us all. I heard an interesting story of parents who were very anti-fluoride, so made sure that the children did not have any fluoride tablets, and lived in an area where there was a negligible amount of fluoride in the water. The children were allowed to use large amounts of toothpaste, however, and when their permanent teeth erupted, there was very distinct evidence of fluoride mottling.

Some toothpastes use stannous fluoride as the active ingredient.

This can cause unsightly staining of the teeth – a worrying prospect if you have been told by the advertisements that toothpaste will make your teeth whiter! I believe that all the ingredients in the formulation of toothpaste should be clearly printed on the container. There should also be a large warning 'Do Not Swallow' (see page 147 for details of ingredients). (Another possible use for toothpaste is to stick children's posters to their bedroom walls. It apparently doesn't leave a mark – or so I'm told!)

FLUORIDE GELS

Many dentists, as part of a preventative regime, will apply a fairly concentrated (approximately 2 per cent) solution, or gel, to the child's developing dentition. This would not normally take place before the age of six as it is important that the patient be old enough to ensure that none of the fluoride is swallowed. This age will coincide with the eruption of the first molar teeth, and these are the teeth which are often heavily filled or lost due to early attacks of tooth decay. If applied to these newly erupted teeth fluoride uptake into the enamel appears to be good and is offering protection at a time when it is most needed. Topical fluoride application can be of benefit at any age, but is especially advantageous between the ages of six and fourteen years. There are adults, however, who are particularly prone to tooth decay and regular applications of topical fluoride can be included in a programme of dietary rehabilitation and oral hygiene techniques. In many dental practices these valuable preventative measures are often undertaken by the hygienist.

Topical fluoride has been found to be of benefit to patients who suffer from sensitive teeth. The concentrated solution appears to provide a form of protection to the sensitive surface.

FLUORIDE MOUTH RINSES

Solutions can be obtained from the chemist in less concentrated form for home use. However, this solution must be treated as a potential poison and consequently should only be used with the explicit instructions of a dentist. It is definitely not suitable for young children. This is a useful method of a regular home-preventative treatment but is normally only prescribed to those whose tooth-decay rate is high. Again, the same safety precautions should be adhered to with regard to home use and storage as with the drops and tablets.

In conclusion, fluoride is found naturally present in the earth's crust, but experiments on animals have shown that if they are totally deprived of fluoride there appears to be no decline in their overall health. This would therefore signify that fluoride is not an essential nutrient. I therefore feel that to introduce fluoride into our bodies is superfluous, and the emphasis should not be on how to increase our bodily intake, but on how to minimize it!

CHAPTER SEVEN

Gum Disease

Gum disease is the most common disease in the world, much more so than the common cold; in fact, there is undeniably *some* stage of the disease, however minor, in every single mouth. Some 98 per cent of the world's population has dental disease of some sort, and about 98 per cent of that percentage in turn is suffering from a clinically recognizable gum disease. It's the principal cause of tooth loss in people over the age of twenty-five, and if it cannot ever entirely be eradicated, as might tooth decay, it could be diminished to an enormous degree by many of the same factors involved in the prevention of tooth decay – good hygiene, regular dental attendances and, once again, diet.

Gum disease is, in fact, much more dangerous than tooth decay. Most decay in teeth can be halted, the teeth can be repaired, and thus the tooth can be saved. However, if gum disease is allowed to develop and progress, it threatens the *foundation* of the teeth, the bone that holds them in the jaw. Once bone loss occurs, the teeth become less secure, and ultimately they too will be lost.

The Function of the Gums

The mouth is a unique part of the human body, for in it occurs the one break in the skin which covers and seals the entire body. Skin stretches over the head, body, feet, fingers – excluding only the eyes perhaps – and even the change from facial skin to the soft moist tissue inside the mouth is only a move from one type of skin to another. Skin stops our insides falling out and stops unwelcome outsiders such as dirt and bacteria getting in. But once teeth are present, there is a junction between the hard mineral – the tooth – and the non-mineralized skin, the gum. There is a *break* in the skin which occurs nowhere else in the body, and this could be the reason why the gums are so vulnerable to disease. Because of that join, they are in a sense a weak link in the overall design of the body.

The principal functions of the gums are to act as a protective covering over the bone holding the teeth, and to hug tightly against teeth to prevent infection reaching that bone. Some people believe that the teeth are set in the gums, but in reality teeth are set in bone, and the gum is merely a security blanket, so to speak. The illustration on the next page will clarify this. And, in order to perform their functions, the gums have many protective factors.

Healthy gums are pink, firm, with a nice clean edge to the scallops where they meet the teeth and go round their contours. The pink colour may be darker in people who are coloured because the gums can contain melanin, the skin mechanism that gives people in hot climates a genetically brown skin, and which browns a white skin when in sun. A healthy gum is stippled like orange peel (only visible when you look very closely): these little holes are where the fibres hold the gums on to the tooth or bone beneath, pulling the gums in rather like the buttoning on a mattress. The gums between the teeth should come to a nice little point, and be the same pale pink colour. These areas often show disease first of all. At the gingival margin – the join line between tooth and gum – there should be no separation or pulling away of gum from the tooth, but this is in theoretical total health. In reality, there is usually a separation of up to 2 mm (less than ⅛ inch), which is still considered good gum health; it is when this minute gap becomes deeper that gum disease is said to be occurring.

As skin sheds dead cells and replaces them with new cells, so do the gums. The cell turnover on the gum is roughly about every 10–12 days; elsewhere in the mouth – on the palate, tongue and cheeks, for instance, where there's more abrasion – the turnover is higher, about every 5–6 days. In the gum crevice, the theoretical 2 mm between gum and tooth, the cell turnover is higher, especially when there is disease present. Then the white defence cells, found in the blood generally, rush to the site of infection and then

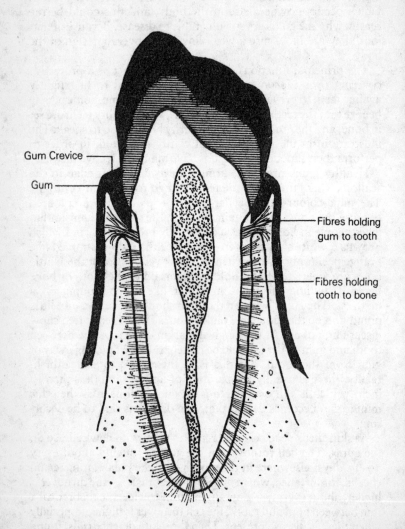

Gum Crevice

Gum

Fibres holding gum to tooth

Fibres holding tooth to bone

Close-up of a healthy tooth

migrate out of the gums into the mouth. The gums exude a fluid, the gingival fluid, which increases during illness, and is also a major defence mechanism. This contains numerous enzymes, those migrating and dead cells, antibodies, immunoglobulins – all the factors we associate with our complex saliva – and indeed the functions of the two are very similar. As saliva is intimately associated with the build-up of plaque, so too are the gum fluids. Indeed the type of plaque and tooth decay can be influenced by the gum fluid. Sub-gingival calculus, for instance, the calculus which forms *under* the gum margin, is usually a blackish colour due to the inclusion of blood from the gum fluid. Just like saliva, the fluid has a washing-away effect, and, in conditions of health and maintenance, the outflow of fluid should be fast and of good quality.

The Causes of Gum Disease

Any disease marks a malfunctioning of the body, and gum disease is no different. If the body is healthy, all the functions of body and mouth will be healthy, the saliva and gingival fluid flow will be healthy, and there should be no gum disease. That all of us show some signs of gum disease is a real indictment of our general health, particularly since there are so many body defence mechanisms to prevent it. The mouth, when considering gum disease, acts as a barometer of health, as an early-warning system, alerting us to deficiencies in the body, and I believe those deficiencies are principally of diet. However, there are often direct and indirect factors which are more generally accepted as the fundamental causes.

PLAQUE
Gum disease first shows itself by an inflammation of the gums which is produced by an accumulation of bacterial plaque near to the gum margins. Any factors which encourage this accumulation, or which prevent its effective removal, will promote and intensify the inflammation. This is the major initial cause of gum disease in theory, but, believe it or not, there is no absolute proof that bacteria and gum disease or periodontal disease are directly

related. However, it is generally accepted that if the bacteria are removed, gum disease doesn't occur; that if the plaque is removed, gum disease doesn't occur. There *is* a relationship, obviously, but it's not the whole answer.

Plaque produces inflammation in the gums in various ways. It is thought that plaque releases histamine and related products from the cells of the gum. This is a defence mechanism of the body generally – the swelling and irritation produced by a nettle sting, say, or allergy. Plaque also directly eats into the gums, which again calls forth inflammation defences. The plaque actually produces poisons which also eat chemically into the gum. All cause swelling, and as soon as this occurs, the crevice is transformed into a pocket within which the bacteria can shelter. All in all, plaque is undoubtedly very destructive to the gums, and the above illustrates very clearly how important brushing the teeth free of plaque is in the control of gum disease. No plaque, no attack on the gums.

OTHER PREDISPOSING FACTORS
These are considered to be many in strict textbook terms, and indeed one factor is thought to be genetic. This predisposition could be racial or familial, but there is absolutely no reason why someone should lose their teeth through gum disease just because a parent did. The vulnerability to the disease may be there genetically, but the disease will still only occur if the circumstances – poor diet and hygiene – enhance it; through *good* diet and hygiene you can still keep your teeth.

Local factors in the mouth. These can predispose to gum disease. If the teeth are awkwardly shaped, with areas where roots have shrunk or been exposed, or crevices, the plaque can be difficult to clean away thoroughly. If teeth are missing, this can start up the process of gum disease: a tooth opposite a missing tooth will continue growing (with nothing to oppose it) and will also tilt. A tilted tooth is very much more difficult to clean than a straight one. If, for example, the top teeth compress food down into gaps between the bottom teeth because of slight tilting or awkward spacing, the food and bacteria can become impacted, causing irritation.

Tooth decay can be a predisposing factor, especially if there is a cavity in close proximity to the gums. A rough cavity is much more difficult to get clean than a smooth surface. If dental fillings don't fit well or if they overlap, it means there are inaccuracies in the joins and, of course, these are wonderful havens for bacteria. So bad dentistry – fillings that don't join properly or two fillings that join together (so that the area between the teeth cannot be cleaned) – can actually predispose to gum disease as well. Sometimes, though, even with good dentistry to start with, the situation can change: if someone has a heavy bite, over the years a metal filling could creep, like lead on a roof, so that it creates an overhang between teeth which will then be difficult to clean.

With crowns, there is always a join line, of course, which will be big enough for the bacteria to settle in. In theory, a crown or filling join line should always be above the gumline so that the toothbrush can brush it clean. On the front teeth, however, for cosmetic reasons, this is not practical. The only answer with any crown, or indeed filling, is to institute and maintain very strict hygiene measures to inhibit food stagnation and plaque formation.

Another factor is bad partial dentures, and in some countries plastic dentures are virtually banned because they are such a major factor in gum disease. These dentures rest on the gums, and as the gums move to chew, the dentures move about on top of them, rubbing and wearing away the surface both of the existing teeth, and of the gum. The denture can also act as a food impaction area: when the food goes on to the denture, it can shed on to the gum area instead of back into the mouth. Indeed the denture can often act just like a piston, thumping the food into areas of gum. Metal dentures are very much more accurate and won't move so much. Dental work of any kind – and this includes braces and other orthodontic appliances – must always be done to the highest possible standards to avoid any encouragement of bacteria and plaque formation.

Direct trauma like sticking a fork prong into the gum can cause gum disease if the area is not kept clean. Biting on the gum flap that occurs when wisdom teeth erupt can also set up the inflammation process. People who breathe through their mouths, or those whose lip closure is inadequate, can suffer inflammation of the gums because of the drying-up effect, with a less efficient flow of cleansing saliva. This affects people with even the most minor nasal problems – such as colds – or those who suffer from ailments like adenoids.

Host factors. I believe that when dealing with gum disease the complete individual has to be considered, and that not to do so is to invite failure. Bacteria and plaque accumulation is a symptom of a generalized body malfunction, as are the results of that accumulation, gum disease and tooth decay.

But dentists in dental schools are not taught to think like this. They are taught half the story – about the gums alone – and never seem to question the missing half – the people to whom those gums belong. A poor salivary flow is a textbook predisposing host factor to gum disease, and should be seen as a generalized relationship between poor salivary flow and the general health of the whole body. Other textbook factors are gums that are softer than they should be, and which therefore do not offer so much protection; a saliva and gingival fluid which are not so rich in protective factors as they should be; poor cell regeneration in the gum crevice; and poor cell secretion of defence mechanisms. All these are symptoms of how the *body* is responding to a situation, and they should never be considered in isolation from that body.

Age is considered a fundamental predisposing factor to gum disease, but it too is looked at in the textbooks purely from the situation in the mouth. Certainly with age, there is a passive eruption of the teeth – in other words, the gums shrink back – but another factor that is quoted is the narrowing of the blood vessels leading to the gums. But this narrowing can be a symptom of age *throughout* the body, of atherosclerosis, etc., another aspect of the whole person. However, time is also a factor here, and irritation that has been chronic for years will have made the whole situation deteriorate progressively.

The sex hormones can predispose to gum disease. I have already mentioned pregnancy gingivitis, but the years of puberty and of the menopause can also be dogged by gum problems. This is true of women on the contraceptive pill as well, who are ingesting hormones, and I always ask female patients – to their occasional surprise – if they are on the pill. Progesterone, oestrogen and testosterone all create a heightened response of the oral tissues to bacteria and plaque. It's not actually disease in itself, and indeed there may be a very low level of bacteria or plaque activity, but the hormones will accelerate and accentuate the normal body responses. This is why it is so important that gum care and health should be an absolute priority at these times, especially during pregnancy which is such an extended period of hormonal change. The free treatment during pregnancy should concentrate, as I've said before in Chapter Three, on gum care and advice, not on tooth decay.

Certain illnesses can cause gum problems. Diabetes, in particular, affects the body responses in general, and there is a great susceptibility to gum disease, to a more rapid bone destruction, and an increased tendency to abscess formation. Blood disorders will also affect the gums. Leukaemia – cancer of the blood – is a classic one, and indeed many childhood leukaemias are first detected by the dentist – an excellent example of how an early screening by the dentist can help. The characteristic signs are swollen bleeding gums, and if a child has had good dental health up till that time, then leukaemia is the first possibility that the dentist will consider. Here, as with diabetes, there is an altered immune response: the immune cells are no longer normal – they are now leukaemic – so there is altered resistance to gum disease.

Diet is mentioned hardly at all in the textbooks as a factor in gum disease, apart from the occasional mention of the relationship between the bleeding gums of scurvy and a lack of Vitamin C. That undergraduate students are encouraged to dismiss the significance of diet is quite beyond my comprehension. One only needs to look at dental history, to refer to the work of Dr Weston Price, to study epidemiological surveys on populations, and the relationship between gum disease and diet stands out in far greater relief than any of the other predisposing factors. When the writers of textbooks claim there is no clear relation between gum disease and diet, whether because they lack sufficient nutritional training to understand it, or simply haven't considered it, I feel both surprised and disappointed.

Diagnosing Gum Disease

Dental confirmation and advice should always be sought as soon as any signs manifest themselves. Fear often prevents dental consultation, but it must be remembered that the sooner treatment is started, the sooner the disease process can be reversed: if it is left, it can only deteriorate, and subsequent treatment, discomfort and eventual health of the mouth will be very much worse. *Never* be afraid to go to the dentist.

THE SIGNS OF GUM DISEASE

If the earliest signs are ignored, the gum crevice separating the gum and the tooth will deepen and the bacterial attack becomes worse. Once the 2 mm of health stretches to even 3 mm, the gum pocket now created can be extremely difficult to keep clean, and if plaque becomes calculus, no home treatment will be effective. The toxins from a pocket of even 4 mm can start to destroy bone, and severe gum disease – periodontitis – has begun. If enough bone is destroyed, the teeth will become loose and will be lost.

Bleeding gums. One of the first questions any dentist should ask a patient, especially a new one, is 'Do your gums bleed?', for *any* bleeding indicates the beginnings of gum disease; and this can occur when brushing, when eating, or with gentle probing. Obviously an accidental bash on the gums which splits the skin will cause bleeding, but the gums should be firm enough to withstand quite rigorous brushing without blood being drawn. As soon as any blood is seen – on the brush, in the spat-out saliva, or the gum itself – this means that there is gum disease present. And bleeding from the gums is so common and becomes so habitual, that most people don't worry about it. It's in these early stages that most can be done by the owner of the gums to alleviate and halt the process, so any bleeding should never be ignored. The adage 'Ignore it and it'll go away' could not be more wrong than when considering gum disease: or, with justification, it could be re-interpreted as, 'Ignore bleeding from the gums and your teeth will go away'. For that initial bleeding of gingivitis or inflammation of the gum can lead, very swiftly, on to the more severe form of gum disease, when bone loss is involved, and when tooth loss is virtually inevitable.

The mouth once again in these early disease stages shows some of its unique properties. It's different from the rest of the body in that it's rare for an infection to cause frank bleeding. If you get an infection elsewhere, there will probably be pus and fluid; in the gums, though, blood is the first sign, and if pus does occur, this means the disease is very severely advanced. Also the action demanded by bleeding in the mouth is quite different from that accorded to bleeding elsewhere in the body. If you have a bleeding area on the hand or leg, say, even a cut lip, the last thing you would want to do is to brush it, poke it and continually wash it: you would want the blood to clot. But in the mouth, if you have bleeding, the last thing you want to do is leave it alone!

To stop bleeding on the gums, the only answer is to brush more, to irrigate more, and generally pay much more attention to the site of the bleeding. Although there may be *more* bleeding at first in response to careful and thorough brushing, the more you brush and irrigate over a period of about twenty-four hours, the less the gum will bleed, and the quicker it will return to normal, clean, healthy tissue. It's a vicious circle, really, and people are conditioned by their instinctive reactions to blood elsewhere in the body: they don't brush their teeth because it makes the gums bleed, but the gums are bleeding because the teeth are not being brushed! To *prevent* gum disease the teeth, in theory, need only be brushed once a day, but once disease is present, the teeth need to be brushed more often.

Red and swollen gums. This is a major sign of gum disease, along with bleeding. Gums will change to red from their normal pink colour, and there will be swelling, especially between the teeth, and tenderness. Any alteration in the appearance, colour or size of gums should be taken seriously, and a dentist's advice should be sought.

Unpleasant taste or bad breath. The taste may be caused by the blood from the gums, of course, or it may be food debris stagnating on the gum or in the gum crevices. This is not an entirely reliable sign because the more the taste is tasted, the less it will be recognized as alien by the taste buds. As with bad breath, individuals may become very quickly accustomed to it, for the same reason; if it persists, though, it is quite often a sign of early gum disease. The characteristic smell of gum disease which every dentist will be able to differentiate from bad breath or food stagnation, is more associated with advanced gum disease. It smells, frankly, of putrefaction.

Receding gums. Disease causes the gums to shrink away from the crowns of the teeth and expose some of the roots. With less support from the gums, the teeth will be very much less secure. Age, as mentioned already, can cause a gum recession not directly associated with gum disease, and this is why older people are said to be 'long in the tooth', for gum recession does inevitably make the teeth look longer. Gums can also shrink back through excessive toothbrushing.

Discomfort and pain. The gums do not usually cause discomfort, but when they do it can be a sign of advanced disease. It only really occurs in acute attacks or if you suddenly decide to brush more thoroughly than usual: if there are severely diseased areas, the brushing can cause discomfort or pain. Vague aching and itching can be symptoms as well. Abscesses can be caused by gum disease and will obviously cause pain. They occur on the side of teeth rather than at the tip of the root, when the contents of the deepened crevice cannot escape into the mouth. Abscesses can severely eat into the supporting bone.

Change of bite. When there is any change in the way that your teeth come together when biting, this means basically that the teeth are starting to move because of bone loss. It is not the *only* cause, for problems with the jaw joints (see page 186) can also make the teeth feel as if they were not meeting properly. But when this change is added to the other signs, it is probably due to fairly advanced gum disease.

Change in partial denture fit. The role of plastic partial dentures in gum disease has already been mentioned. When they cease to fit properly, it means that the position of teeth in the gums has altered, and the gum itself will be shrinking back.

Pus. Pus is the sign of a severe infection in any part of the body, and particularly in the mouth. Dental advice must be sought as soon as possible and treatment instituted immediately. It can show yellow between the teeth, and can come out of the gums when you press on them.

Loose or separating permanent teeth. Unless you are between six and twelve, when you might expect to have wobbly teeth, any looseness is caused by gum disease. This is when the foundation bone has been severely eroded, and inflammation may extend over most of the root of the tooth. Once this extends round the end of the root, the tooth will fall out. If the teeth are also separating, however slightly, it means that they're actually drifting apart as well as loosening. It is very sad on front teeth, where it's commonly seen; they spread apart, and one incisor may be longer than the other. The body is almost starting to reject the teeth; it doesn't want them there any more. This is severe gum disease, and purely conventional treatment – even scaling every six weeks – will not be truly effective.

The progress of gum disease

Warning Signs	Stage of Gum Disease
1 Bleeding gums	Early sign
2 Red, swollen or tender gums	Early sign in most cases
3 Bad breath and bad taste	Early or advanced
4 Receding gums	Early or advanced
5 Discomfort and pain	Usually advanced
6 Change of bite	Advanced
7 Change in partial denture fit	Advanced
8 Pus	Bad advanced
9 Loose or separating teeth	Severe advanced

ACUTE GUM DISEASE

Most gum disease is chronic in that it can rumble on for ages before showing any clinical symptoms. However, children from puberty onwards, from about twelve to twenty, can develop an acute, or very rapidly progressing, condition known as juvenile periodontitis. It is associated with periods of severe gum infection and areas of severe bone loss around the teeth. It is treated as gum disease in general with mouthwashes and intensive gum therapy, but it is a classic instance of where the *whole person* should be considered. As far as diet is concerned, this is a bad age, but it is also a time of great stress: pressures are put on at school, exams come round with unremitting regularity, and the emotional traumas and body changes of puberty can be stressful as well. Little research has been undertaken on these aspects, despite the fact that there would seem to be a very logical association.

Another stress-related condition is called variously acute ulcerative gingivitis, Vincent's infection or trench mouth. The gums are sore, red and bleeding, and ulcers and pus are often present. It develops very rapidly, and is sometimes thought to be contagious (it's not) because it affects people in groups: men in the trenches suffered it because of the triple combination of poor diet, bad hygiene and stress. Nowadays it afflicts people who, under stress, get it suddenly, out of the blue, when there are severe emotional strains. It is a time when antibiotics like metronidazole and tetracycline are very useful.

OTHER MOUTH CONDITIONS

Not all are gum disease, but many of the signs could look the same. Some chemicals such as aspirin can cause burns and ulcerations (when an aspirin is held, say, close to an aching gum or tooth). Ulcers or cold sores can develop from viruses such as herpes, both inside and outside the mouth, and the thrush virus can cause soreness and irritation. Some drugs can cause a sensitivity reaction in the mouth, with swelling, soreness and ulcers. The eruption of the wisdom teeth, as already mentioned, can cause inflammation and ultimate infection.

Mouth ulcers – aphthous ulcers – are very common, occurring in some 40–50 per cent of the population. They are painful, worrying (in that it is a breakdown in the skin for no apparent reason), and they can and do recur. Nutritional deficiencies could be one cause, and the amount of ulceration could be reduced by giving chlorhexedine mouthwashes, certain vitamins, the B complex and C in particular, and some minerals such as zinc.

Any mouth condition which worries should be seen by a dentist.

THE ROLE OF THE DENTIST

In diagnosing gum disease and treating it, the dentist must play an enormous role. By concentrating on gum disease advice and care, he will truly be saving teeth – which is what he's there for. Thirty years ago, the dread word 'pyorrhoea' (an old-fashioned word for disease of the mouth, not used often by the profession) would have meant extraction, but now, with our far wider knowledge, gum disease can be halted and teeth can be saved. I cannot emphasize enough how important it is for a dentist to be consulted regularly, and as soon as any signs of the disease become apparent.

Although home brushing can often cope with the first bleeding signs, the dentist should be made aware of the situation. He can advise on brushing: as gums can literally heal within hours, a soft brush and a thorough and careful brushing will remove the first layers of plaque, and the gums can reduce in size. He can advise on reaching difficult areas, and start the process off himself. However swollen and painful the gums are, he can gently scale the teeth, slipping the scaler in between tooth and gum to clean the tooth and remove the plaque and calculus; thereafter the gingival fluids should wash away the infection. The basic point is that the more you can do while the infection or inflammation is there – whether at home by brushing, or with a scaling from the dentist – the quicker the disease will go away. The dentist and his diagnosis are the first line of defence.

Nutrition and Gum Disease

When first considering the relationship between the two, it should be remembered that gum disease relates entirely to living tissue, and therein lies its major difference from tooth decay. It could be argued that a tooth is living, but in fact its surface layer is inert, with no nerve endings or blood supply. Tooth decay can respond with remineralization, with fluoride, etc. – an indirect response – but gum disease is related totally to tissue that can respond directly. It concerns a direct response mechanism from living tissue, and therefore gum disease is entirely related to the host response. This is why, of course, gum disease can begin so much more rapidly than tooth decay. Although an acidic attack on a tooth can begin within minutes, the tooth will not suffer technical damage for months: in twenty-four hours, though, because of poor resistance, the initial stages of gum disease can become quite severe.

I've discussed already the host factors generally considered to lead to gum disease, and my own theories, and I do feel that nutrition must be the major one. Because host resistance to disease is affected by health, and health is affected by nutrition, gum disease must have a relationship to nutrition. Although there was an upsurge of interest in nutrition in the twenties and thirties, since then the subject has not been explored in any great depth either in research or in the textbooks. The emphasis has been on the treatment of disease rather than on the causes, and although treatment is obviously vital, it's a rather blinkered situation. Why *is* dental disease more prevalent now despite these advances in science and all these treatments? Could it not be due to faulty nutrition? Could it not be due also to environmental stresses – more severe now than thirty years ago – and personal stresses? Research has got to take into account the *people* who suffer from disease, and only by looking at them – how they eat, what they eat, how they live, how they cope in general – can proper evaluations and judgements be made.

Disease is always a multi-factorial situation – it can never be put down to *one* cause alone, for why then do only a percentage of those who smoke contract lung cancer? – so if environmental stresses cannot be altered, and personal emotional stresses are difficult to counteract, good diet would seem to be a major way in which body resistance to disease can be boosted directly and easily. A good wholefood diet which will boost general health will undoubtedly *help* in the fight against gum disease. Indeed, one of the host factors mentioned in textbooks as contributing to gum disease is the lack of function involved in eating soft pappy and mushy foods. This also relates to the incidence of tooth decay, of course, in that whole, hard foods are more likely to have a detergent action, and with the whole jaw moving more, more saliva being brought into play, the plaque, the initiator of gum disease, will be less likely to get a hold.

However, in a less general sense, there are certain dietary factors that are believed to help in the fight against gum disease. Vitamin C, for instance, was potent against scurvy – the main symptoms of which were bleeding gums – and therefore increased Vitamin C levels can help regenerate tissue and boost resistance. Vitamin C can be diminished in the body by things like smoking (some gum specialists will not treat patients if they continue smoking), by the pill, by fevers and, perhaps astonishingly, by aspirin. If someone has a painful gum disease and they take aspirin, the Vitamin C levels of the body can be reduced to a level as low as that found in severe scurvy; if that aspirin were held against the gum to prevent pain, the ulceration from aspirin burn can make the situation doubly worse.

Vitamin C is the main nutritional factor to be directly related to gum disease, but the other minerals found in a good diet will all help balance the situation. Lack of zinc and calcium, and too much phosphorus, are thought to be associated with bone loss. The latter two are directly associated with eating too much meat, and one 'type' of sufferer from gum disease does appear to me, from clinical practice, to be the expense-account lunch eater, who will be eating rich and heavy protein foods. Athletes too, who eat a great deal of protein for muscle building, could, ironically, have calcium and zinc deficiencies as a result, which will contribute to gum disease.

Most of us do have gum disease, and it's unlikely, unless we all change to a 100 per cent wholefood diet, and can clean our teeth with 100 per cent efficiency, that this situation will radically change. Remember that gum disease is a *repeatable* disease; a perfect diet and perfect cleaning one week will do wonders, but the gum disease will come back if the regime is not continued. What we have to look at for the long-term future, is the rate of *progress* of the disease. If it's slow, then teeth could be rock-solid even after a lifetime – something we would all want. So, if we can't be perfect, we should work towards a lowering of the incidence, a slowing down of the progress of the disease, and a boosting of the individual resistance to the disease. In this way, we might still suffer signs of the disease, but would not be troubled by it. This, then, must be the priority of every dentist, medical researcher, nutritionist, and vulnerable patient.

CHAPTER EIGHT

Keeping Your Mouth Clean

If you've read in the previous chapters of all the bacterial activity in the mouth, of the speed at which plaque can form, and of the speed at which the initial stages of both tooth decay and gum disease can develop, then it will be obvious why it is vital to keep your mouth clean. Oral hygiene is the most direct way in which plaque can be combated by every individual, whether he or she be six months old or ninety years old. Although I don't believe, sadly, that anyone can ever guarantee to be 100 per cent efficient, any cleaning at all will help diminish the attacks by disease – so why not aim to do the very best possible in the cause of a healthy mouth and sound teeth and gums. It may be a chore, but the amount of time you spend every day keeping your mouth clean is one of the best investments you can make for health and lasting good looks.

Toothbrushing

This is the key to plaque control, for plaque cannot be *washed* off the teeth, it must be abraded or brushed off. Brushing is also the most natural process of cleaning your teeth: it does not introduce any chemicals, it does not upset the balance of the oral flora, it does not involve the ingestion of anything that might be harmful – it just literally breaks down any established plaque and disorganizes it. If you brush several times a day, plaque will not basically be given the chance to settle anywhere, and thus you will be severely impeding the progress of both tooth decay and gum disease.

The number of times you should brush per day depends really

on how thorough your brushing is. To be safe, though, to prevent tooth decay, you should brush after every meal: in fact, as already mentioned, to prevent the possibility of plaque reaction with sugars in a meal, teeth could be brushed free of plaque *before* a meal. Twice a day – after breakfast, and before going to bed – are generally enough, but not if sugary snacks are eaten between meals. This is the danger time when saliva flow is low and the bacterial count is highest. To prevent gum disease, it is only really necessary to brush once a day, in theory; once gum disease has developed, in however minor a form, as already stated, more frequent gentle brushing is vital to get rid of accumulated plaque and bring the gums back to normal.

HOW TO BRUSH YOUR TEETH

All dentists agree that home brushing is a major factor in plaque control, but I believe the dentist could involve himself even further: he should look at the brushing technique of each and every one of the patients when they are in the surgery. Only then can he see, perhaps, the areas they are missing and that are therefore vulnerable to attack; only then can he correct a faulty technique, or advise a better one. Even if all the dentist does on a patient's first visit is give basic brushing instructions, the patient can see and feel a dramatic difference in mouth health – especially if they have an established gum disease – in no more than forty-eight hours. This has a dual benefit: it shows the patient what can be done – all for the cost of a toothbrush – and it makes the dentist appear a virtual miracle worker in the patient's eyes! When time is spent giving instructions on how to brush, patients say their mouths feel much cleaner and healthier thereafter. A feedback like this is vital for a dentist, and it is fundamental for the whole relationship between dentist and patient: if he has managed to improve the situation, in however minor a way, the patient will feel better and more positive about his mouth and teeth, knowing he can do so much for himself.

Modes of brushing do vary and they tend to go through fashions: at one time it was up and down, then it was from side to side . . . and it's no wonder that people get confused. However, as I've emphasized throughout the book, even here the method will have to be individual because the mouth and teeth of all of us are individual. Everyone has teeth and jaws of different shapes and sizes, so the ideal cleaning techniques will differ. This is where individual tuition must come in, and it should be a major function of the dentist and his team, the dental educator and the dental hygienist.

The main movement, though, is a sort of small rotary action, in which the gum and tooth are massaged together, with the brush held at an angle of about 45 degrees to the tooth. Cover only two or three teeth at a time so that you don't miss any. Many people find it more convenient to clean the back surfaces of their teeth with the brush pointing into the mouth lengthways, especially at the front where the dental arch is most curved. Finally, clean the biting surfaces by using the rotary action firmly over all the molars and the teeth in front, upper and lower, to clean out any crevices and fissures thoroughly.

The movement should be firm, but not too hard; as I've said before, too vigorous brushing can actually damage the tooth enamel and can make the gums shrink back, exposing the cementum and dentine. The final step is to rinse the mouth out thoroughly with cold water.

Try to brush your teeth in front of a mirror so that you can see what you are doing, and that the brush is going where it ought to. Although brushing should become a habit almost from the word go, as soon as the deciduous teeth erupt, it can become *too* much of a habit sometimes. This is when an area might habitually be missed, and dentists see this often, usually around the canines, left or right, depending on which hand the brusher uses. The dentist or hygienist will be able to correct this when they watch you cleaning in the surgery, but one way round it might be to deliberately change the pattern and order of your brushing every now and then to ensure that all the teeth are covered.

TOOTHBRUSHES

Although twigs and bristles were used in the past for toothpicks and for brushing the teeth, the modern toothbrush probably evolved only fairly recently, in the eighteenth century. It is said to have been invented by William Addis, a stationer whose name became attached to the household brush company. In hiding after the Gordon Riots in 1780, Addis hid in a slaughterhouse where he whiled away the hours by carving bone. He then had the brilliant idea of boring small holes in one end of a bone handle and inserting horsehair into them. This, then, was the fairly inauspicious origin of the first toothbrush! Since then the toothbrush has been refined and modified – with handles of celluloid, then plastic; with bristles of natural bristle, then nylon – and the industry has flourished. Britain is apparently one of the top three consumers of toothbrushes per capita in the world, but it is also a virtually static consumption. Despite recommendations from dentists that brushes should be replaced every four to six weeks (two to three months at the longest), the average adult buys only 1.25 brushes per year – around 56 million brushes in 1984.

The dentist should be consulted about the type of brush to use, for again individual instruction is needed. There are literally about a hundred types of toothbrush design on the market, with varying sizes, types of bristle, and lengths of handle, and all these can influence how well the toothbrush is used. In general, though, the surround of the head – the part in which the bristles are set – should be smooth and rounded so that nothing can jar against tissues in the mouth, and the head itself should be fairly small. With a large head, you could probably sweep over about four teeth at a time, missing small areas; with a small head you can more painstakingly concentrate on each tooth. The bristle should be of nylon, not of natural bristle – and this is one 'unnatural' introduction to the mouth. Natural bristle has got larger filaments than nylon, and the ends are cut during the manufacturing process: if the massaging method of cleaning is used with natural bristles this sharp cut-off end can microscopically cut the gums. Nylon filaments have ends which are rounded and polished. They are also designed specifically to be soft enough to bend and flex into the 2 mm gum crevice of theoretical perfect health. Toothbrush filaments should be hard enough to remove plaque but soft enough so that they don't damage the gum; really hard brushes aren't necessary. The dentist or hygienist will be able to advise on the number of bristle rows needed on the brush head. This again relates to the size of mouth and teeth.

Many dentists do now sell toothbrushes, and they should ideally carry a range of various manufacturers' wares *and* a range of sizes. I truly believe that just as you need to be fitted by the optician for the right lenses and the right size of frame, so you need to be fitted by the dentist with the right toothbrush. It's not much use being told just the manufacturer's name: there are so many variations. The dentist should also look at how the patient holds the brush, which may indicate a different length of handle: some people with larger hands may need a longer handle (just as they feel happier with a longer-handled table knife). If this concept were taken further, some people suffering from arthritis, say, who can only close their hands to a certain degree, might find holding a thin-handled brush virtually impossible. As a recent dental paper suggested, the dentist could put some soft wax around the handle of a conventional brush and take a mould of the patient's grip, which could then be reproduced in plastic. A simple solution like this could revolutionize the tooth-cleaning technique of many older patients – and their lives.

Many manufacturers are now designing their toothbrush handles with heads of flexi-plastic. This means that the head can be modified – actually bent by the user – to get an angle which is more appropriate to a particular area of the jaw. This idea could do away with the need to buy several brushes for several jobs.

Take care of your brush, and it will last longer. Don't use warm water to dampen it as this will soften the nylon and may permanently distort it. Don't use desperately cold water either, as this could set your teeth on edge. Wash it after use to get rid of any debris, and knock it lightly against the side of the basin to get rid of excess water. Store it upright in a wall-hung tray preferably, so that it can drain properly; if stored in a cup or jar, water will drain into that and will go stale.

Do try to change your brush several times a year. Normally I would say every month or six weeks, but it varies from person to person. When the bristles start to splay, they will not reach into the gum crevice, so that is the time for a change. If you brush your teeth as instructed by the dentist, and you find a brush splays after about a week or so, it might be worth complaining to the manufacturer or trying out another brand to see if that lasts any longer.

Thorough brushing is all that is needed for healthy teeth and gums – for toothpaste isn't strictly necessary – so there's no excuse not to carry a brush with you at all times, in pocket or handbag:

small fold-up travelling brushes are available. And indeed I have seen machines that dispense disposable brushes already pasted: this is a really positive and social step (instant sweet breath), so why aren't they more widely available, in restaurants etc., to cater for that undoubted need?

OTHER BRUSHING AIDS

The conventional type of electric toothbrush, which swirls up and down, is useful for patients who have impaired manual dexterity – arthritics for instance – and also for those who might lack motivation: it's a gadget, quite fun, and no effort because all the work is done for them. Children like that sort of thing too. They're just as good as the conventional toothbrush – but only on nice straight teeth. If there are nooks and crannies, and gums are recessed or roots exposed, that swirling action will not be nearly as effective.

Rotary toothbrushes, which are usually operated by a rechargeable battery, are rather like the polisher a dentist uses. They have a small cup brush with a tapered top which can work in between the teeth. The rotary action ensures a thorough cleaning, and they are particularly good for people who wear dental appliances such as braces. They are relatively expensive, though, and need explicit instructions from the dentist for their use.

Water picks are now available to the public and they are a useful adjunct to brushing in that they can syringe food debris out of the gaps between teeth. They are particularly of value when the gums have shrunk so much that the roots are exposed in arch shapes: conventional methods would not work so well here. The jet is usually strong enough to clean plaque off as well, but not so strong that it harms tissue. They too are expensive, but for selected patients, water picks can generally improve their cleaning efficiency.

Toothpastes

Toothpastes, despite the multi-million pound industry that has grown up around them, are not as essential as one is led to believe. It is the brushing action that is valuable and has the main detergent effect. In most cases the only benefit of toothpaste is the fresh taste it gives, and in some cases toothpastes can be actively harmful in that they can be *too* abrasive. In reality, one could use baking soda, salt or nothing at all! The first proprietory tooth cleaners were powders, and it was not until the beginning of this century, when the collapsible tube was invented, that viscous toothpaste was able to be formulated, packaged and sold.

WHAT'S IN YOUR TOOTHPASTE?
Various factors go to make up the formulations of modern toothpastes. The *polishing agents* are mild abrasives such as dicalcium phosphate, insoluble sodium metaphosphate and chalk (calcium carbonate); the *foaming agents* are detergents; *humecants* such as glycerine and sorbitol keep the paste moist; *binding agents* hold the ingredients of the paste together; the *flavouring agents* are generally blue, pink or white food colourings. Some toothpastes are said to contain mouthwash formulations in their stripes, and some toothpastes actually contain sugar!

Fluoride is added to most toothpastes these days – about 98 per cent of them – and this is undoubtedly responsible for the decrease in tooth decay, especially in our new generation of children. A new enzyme toothpaste has appeared fairly recently on the market, and it does appear to reduce the rate of plaque build-up.

Although toothpaste is not ingested – or should not be – holistic dentists feel that the ingredients of toothpaste should be listed on the packs, as food manufacturers are obliged now to do. It's not a food obviously, but it's sold and bought as one in a sense. I have detailed a few ingredients above – taken from a manufacturer's leaflet – but there are still grey areas. What are the detergents used, what binding agents are used, and in what form are the flavourings? Many of the ingredients used in toothpastes are in quite strong chemical form, and could cause allergic or other reactions, so we feel that the public should be aware of the detailed contents of something they put in their mouths as regularly as foods. Some food colourings are thought to be dangerous, for instance; chlorhexedine, a strong mouthwash, is used in some formulations and not only can that upset the oral flora, it can occasionally *stain* the teeth (so, although you're using the paste to make your teeth white, you could actually be making them worse).

However, when you consider how many toothpastes are manufactured, and how much is sold and used, it is amazing that there is so *little* reaction. But reaction there has been in a few cases, which illustrates that attention does need to be paid to the contents of the formulations. Even if the paste is not directly swallowed, a certain amount inevitably leaches into the tissues of the mouth, or clings to the teeth when not thoroughly rinsed and can be swallowed thereafter. Even 'natural' toothpastes can contain natural allergens. It is children whom I consider most at risk here: they forget, and swallow, and any extra ingestion of fluoride, say, could be harmful. Any reaction of any sort which is thought to be attributable to a toothpaste should be reported to the manufacturer so that it can be monitored and assessed. With the toothpaste market standing at some 93 million pounds in 1985, some of the profits could very profitably be put to researching and producing the best possible toothpastes which will contain ingredients which are totally non-allergic, non-irritant and non-toxic. The manufacturers have done well so far, but I believe they could still do better.

WHICH TOOTHPASTE TO USE

Patients are always asking their dentists for a recommendation and often they will simply be given samples of what the dentist has been sent by the manufacturers. However, there is little difference between them, apart from those containing fluoride, and perhaps those containing enzymes. They must not be swallowed though, so when to be used by a child, the dentist and parent will have to take that into consideration.

Some toothpastes are more abrasive than others, and I cannot recommend the smoker's tooth powder for general use. They might however help someone on drugs which are causing staining. In fact, a toothpaste that becomes progressively *less* abrasive as you brush is perhaps a direction in which the manufacturers might look. It could start off relatively abrasive to clean off the initial layers of plaque, but as you continue to brush, it should become finer in order to give the teeth a good polish. The advantages would be two-fold: the teeth would be very much smoother after brushing, but also, *knowing* that this effect was taking place, people would tend to spend much longer on brushing their teeth – and that is always desirable!

Coloured or striped toothpastes are really a bit of a gimmick, I believe, and most dentists would advise that a white paste is used: as you spit out the foam and saliva, any blood from the gums can be easily seen.

For people with sensitive teeth, I would recommend the de-sensitizing toothpastes, for they seem to work. They too contain chemicals, of course, but their undoubted benefits healthily out-weigh any potential irritation – and indeed their greater cost and their unpleasant taste!

How much toothpaste should you use? As little as possible is the simple answer. The manufacturers are to blame here, as they illustrate their wares in great profitable wodges on a brush: not only is this unnecessary, wasteful and perhaps hazardous, it will foam up to an enormous degree and you won't be able to see what you are doing. A tiny squeeze of paste is all that is necessary for babies, children and adults alike. This is probably the main disadvantage of the new dispensers which give out a measured dose.

Flossing

Most dentists agree that the two best dental treatments are brushing and flossing. Indeed brushing is only half the cleaning story, as the floss is vital for getting into the spaces between the teeth where even the most sensitive and sophisticated brush filaments cannot reach. In theory, with good brushing and good flossing, you could almost achieve 100 per cent efficiency in cleaning. In practice, however, there are problems, and flossing can have its disadvantages. The major benefit of flossing, how-ever, apart from its cleaning power, is that it familiarizes you with your own mouth. It's only through the use of floss that you can become intimate with the geography of your mouth: with the number of teeth, with the spaces, with the nooks and crannies, with the places where food becomes trapped. Once you start to use floss and do so regularly, your mouth and teeth will become part of your body, no longer a mere orifice and chewing instrument for food, and you can build up a special relationship. Fanciful perhaps, but infinitely valuable, and only floss can encourage it.

HOW TO FLOSS YOUR TEETH

Working in front of a mirror, take about 45–60 cm (18–24 inches) of floss and wind each end around the middle finger of each hand, leaving about 15 cm (6 inches) between the fingers. Tighten the floss between thumb and forefinger. Gently guide the floss between two teeth until you touch the gum and feel a gentle pressure. The floss will look as though it's penetrating the gum, but it will be going into the crevice and disorganizing any plaque there. Pull the floss into a 'C' shape around the side of one tooth. Gently guide the floss down or up the tooth in a wiping motion, away from the gum, and then do the same with the other tooth. Wind on some fresh floss with your fingers, and repeat the procedure between every gap, on every tooth. Flossing does undoubtedly require a fair amount of manual dexterity, but with practice you will soon become more adept.

TYPES OF FLOSS

Floss comes in waxed or unwaxed rolls, in pre-cut lengths, or as a plastic tape, and it can be used in the hands or in special flossers. Waxed tape, which is normally wider, could be useful for the first-time user, or for children; it runs between the teeth more easily, and there's less likelihood of fraying; it also tends to be more hygienic as it doesn't get permeated with plaque. Because the unwaxed floss is *not* coated, it will go between very fine gaps, and it will splay to cover a wider area. Flossers, which are becoming more popular, are by far the easiest way of using floss.

THE DISADVANTAGES OF FLOSS

Flossing can show up faulty dentistry. If there are ledges or overhangs on fillings or teeth, the floss will find them out. If the floss frays on these ledges or a rough edge of a crown, it can get caught and can be a source of irritation in itself. If floss is used wrongly, it can cut into the gums and damage them, and an incorrect see-sawing movement might even wear the tooth away at the gumline. If there is a large chunk of food caught between teeth, floss can sometimes push the food further in (using a wood point or toothpick gently, might be a good idea before flossing). However, every cloud has a silver lining, and if floss does reveal faults such as the above, the dentist can be informed and they can be corrected.

Disclosing Tablets

These should be used in conjunction with brushing and flossing as a major factor in combating plaque. They are composed of a vegetable dye, usually 4 per cent erythrosin, and there is a flavouring agent as well. As with anything else to be used in the mouth, they should be — and probably are — non-toxic, non-allergic and non-irritant. They work on the principle that they stain the plaque layer (blue or pink usually), and some are quite sophisticated in that they stain in different shades depending on the thickness of the plaque.

The tablets should be used once a week to check on the general plaque control. The teeth should be brushed and flossed in the normal way then one tablet should be chewed, mixed with saliva, and then gently swished around the teeth. The solution should then be spat out and the mouth rinsed with water. The teeth will show stained areas in the mirror, and these remaining areas of plaque should be brushed off thoroughly.

Mouthwashes

The most natural, and sometimes the most effective, mouthwash is a solution of salty water, and this is particularly useful in reducing oral infections such as gum disease. As much salt as possible should be dissolved in a tumbler full of hot or warm water and then the water taken into the mouth, held over the inflammation for as long as possible, then gargled around the mouth before spitting out. The concentrated salt acts osmotically to draw some of the pus and fluid out of the tissues so that there is less inflammation. It isn't much good for mouth ulcers, though, as it will make them sting.

Proprietary mouthwashes can serve a useful purpose, but most are antiseptic and antibacterial and thus could unbalance the oral flora if used too frequently. Holistically, I would not recommend their use except when advised by a dentist.

A mouthwash that is gaining favour with periodontal or gum disease experts is chlorhexedine which can also be used in home care. Chlorhexedine does undoubtedly work in a number of ways, but it has its disadvantages too. The chemicals in it suppress the oral bacteria, inhibit plaque and calculus formation, and can even dissolve plaque. On the debit side, however, the balance of the oral flora is severely disturbed, and it also causes staining on the teeth, it has an unpleasant taste, and suppresses the taste buds. Again, you should seek expert dental advice. It should be used only in severe disease or in circumstances where other cleaning methods are difficult to institute or monitor, as with the handicapped, say.

Chlorhexedine also seems to help reduce the size and duration of aphthous ulcers – although not their incidence.

Toothpicks and Wood Points

Toothpicks come in all shapes, sizes and materials: the rich use gold, the Chinese use ivory or plastic, the smart set use cocktail sticks, and the needy or desperate use the ends of matches. None will really do an efficient job of plaque removal as they will not curve round the convexity of the tooth. Many will be effective in digging out a large lump of food, but I dread to think of what damage could also be done to fillings or gums. Proprietary wood points can be effective, though, as they are soft and are usually sensibly shaped; areas of food trapping can be relieved, although they are not a great deal of use in plaque control.

These are the broad outlines of how you can cure yourself at home, getting rid of plaque which is the main causative factor of both tooth decay and gum disease. There are certain things only a dentist and his team can do – getting rid of calculus, for instance – but the main emphasis of holistic prevention depends on you, your motivation and your perseverance.

CHAPTER NINE

Dentistry Today

Dentistry today is a specialist science, and every general dental practitioner is a highly skilled professional who has undergone a long and intensive training. The image of the dentist as a tooth-puller has changed dramatically in a comparatively short time, and dentists have gone on to the offensive: their practice is now oriented towards prevention and restoration. Advances in research and material science have given dentists the weapons with which they can achieve these aims.

There has been a lot of controversy recently over how often one should visit the dentist, but I unequivocally recommend the six-monthly interval as the ideal. The significance of that six months is perhaps arbitrary, but in practice, within that time-scale, the progress of disease can be monitored and checked. It is unlikely that we would see new cavities occurring at such frequent intervals, but gum disease, which can develop much more rapidly, often requires an even more frequent professional appraisal. And, of course, because the mouth is a barometer of health, frequent inspection may reveal early sign of systemic disease.

Fillings

The dentist of today is inextricably associated with fillings, but most people do not realize the difficulties he and the profession have had in finding materials that will survive the hostile environment of the mouth. As yet, there is still no ideal solution.

The first requirement of a dental material is that it should not dissolve. The mouth, as already described, is extremely active both bacteriologically and chemically, and most materials – iron, for example – would probably corrode in a matter of days. Secondly, a restoration material must have immense strength, as the force involved in biting can be measured in terms of tons per square inch! This pressure and these stresses would be inflicted on the material day in, day out, and year after year. Also, the vast temperature changes that occur in the mouth have to be considered. For, as with any material, the tooth will contract and expand as the temperature rises or falls, and any material must exhibit a similar property. The difference between an ice-cream one minute and a hot cup of tea the next can cause a temperature change of some fifty degrees centigrade, and any discrepancies in the rates of expansion can lead to gaps and stresses occurring between the tooth and the filling material.

AMALGAM AND THE MERCURY DEBATE
Ideally, we should like any dental materials to be non-irritant to the mouth and non-toxic to the rest of the body. Many dental materials, however, are less than satisfactory in this respect. There is concern, for instance, over the safety of using 'amalgam' fillings – the most common material used for fillings today – in that they contain approximately 50 per cent mercury, a known toxic metal. Much confusion has been generated by recent publications, which have fuelled *unfounded* fears that any severe illness or slight malaise is caused by mercury poisoning, the source being the fillings present in the mouth. I believe that there is no smoke without fire, and thus I feel that medical and dental scientists would be failing in their duty if *thorough* and unbiased research and investigations were not undertaken, using the most widespread terms of reference. It may be the case that potential dangers have not been recognized because they were not looked for. Lead is a classic example. This, another toxic metal as we all now know, is emitted in car fumes, but until recently there was little concern. Having recognized the dangers, researchers found that children living near very busy main roads often had certain disturbances including lower levels of intelligence. Now there is action throughout the world to reduce levels of lead in petrol.

There is no doubt that hundreds of millions of people are walking around today, between them carrying several billion fillings, and the vast majority of them are not keeling over with mercury toxicity. The weight of evidence appears to suggest that if a person has *unexplained* disease or malfunction of the body, then all possible causes must be investigated. If there were, for example, some 100 possible causes, then mercury toxicity would have very low priority, and perhaps as many as ninety other suspects would need to be considered before mercury. In other countries such as Sweden, the mercury debate has been in the public eye for at least ten years, and there are many discussions in the media and even at governmental level. The experience of experts in Scandinavia is that in the vast majority of cases, when people feel they may have mercury toxicity, their fears are largely unfounded. However, every case is taken seriously and thoroughly investigated.

The situation in Great Britain at present is less clear. In answer to a Parliamentary Question in the House of Commons, Health Minister Barney Hayhoe said on 22 October 1985, and I quote from *Hansard*:

'Dental amalgam has been widely used in this and many other countries for over a century to fill cavities in teeth – over 25 million such treatments were provided under the general dental service in England and Wales in 1983 alone, but very few adverse reactions in patients to amalgam have been reported. Most have been an allergic or sensitivity reaction to mercury which is one of the constituents of amalgam and such patients can have their teeth filled with other materials. I am advised that there is no good scientific evidence which would indicate that any clinically significant amounts of mercury are absorbed by patients from fillings in their teeth. Moreover any small degree of risk has to be offset against the substantial benefits of a material which has been proved to be long lasting, convenient for dentists to use and can be produced at relatively low cost. No other modern material has yet been proved as suitable and convenient for most fillings where appearance is not a consideration.

'The potential risk to dentists and their staff from the mishandling of mercury in dental practice is well recognized and can be minimized by taking adequate precautions. Guidelines on the safe handling of mercury prepared by the British Dental Association were last revised and issued in the autumn of 1982.

'Whilst there is therefore no convincing evidence of any obvious health effect on the vast majority of patients, nevertheless it is helpful to have a comprehensive review of the evidence from time to time. For this reason I have asked the Committees on Toxicity and on Dental and Surgical Materials to consider the evidence on the risks and benefits and to let me have their advice in due course.'

Earlier, on 17 October, the British Dental Association issued a five-point statement which could be used as a basis for dentists to answer patients' enquiries in the surgery:

'1 The BDA believes that it is misleading and potentially cruel to suggest to patients, in the absence of a responsible diagnosis, that their neurological symptoms may be cured by extensive, and probably expensive, dental treatment. The BDA advises any dentist considering the replacement of amalgam fillings under these circumstances *not* to undertake this work without obtaining the advice of a consultant neurologist.

'2 Should any patients feel they have an unexplained illness that might be associated with amalgam fillings, they should seek the advice of their doctor or dentist in the first instance. On no account should any patient seek the complete removal of amalgam fillings without consulting expert medical opinion first.

'3 Amalgam has been used in the UK for over a century. Over the ten-year period 1973–1983, some 280 million fillings have been given to patients without evidence of detrimental effects to their overall health. All amalgam preparations used by NHS general dental practitioners in the UK are strictly controlled and approved by the DHSS.

'4 A thorough survey of the scientific literature about mercury toxicity reveals that there is *no* substantiated evidence of neurological symptoms at the mercury levels that could arise from amalgam fillings. There are a few reports of allergic reactions but these are extremely rare. Any such reactions occur quickly and a diagnosis may be easily confirmed. A similar conclusion is reached in a recently published review of the world literature on mercury toxicity.

'5 The BDA welcomes all scientific research into existing dental materials and into the development of new alternatives. The safety of patients must remain paramount. At the present time there is no satisfactory alternative to amalgam for certain types of fillings and no reason to discontinue its use.'

Strong words of reassurance from both Government and the BDA, which is the official body representing a large proportion of the nation's dentists. I would agree, largely, with this responsible, if pedantic, point of view.

It appears ironic that nearly 150 years ago the American Dental Association excluded all dentists who used mercury fillings from membership and labelled them charlatans. As the only viable alternative for filling teeth was gold, mercury fillings gradually became accepted, primarily on the grounds of low cost and ease of use. Today's amalgam fillings are more refined than those of 100 years ago, but are still very similar in composition. There are two main constituents of amalgam: pure mercury, which at room temperature is liquid, silver in colour and, if placed on a flat surface, produces distinct globules; and the alloy, which is a grey powder composed of silver (approximately 65 per cent), tin (approximately 25 per cent), and other metals such as copper and zinc in much smaller amounts. The mercury and alloy are mixed together in approximately equal proportions. This is normally carried out by a machine which will vibrate the constituents to ensure an even mix. The outcome is a stiff grey paste and, from a dentist's point of view, is ideal for placing into a tooth cavity and for consequent contouring and carving. Most amalgams take about twenty-four hours to fully harden, and when polished they will develop a high silvery lustre which could rival any highly polished car! So what is all the fuss about?

It was generally believed that once the amalgam had set there would be no further reaction and that there would be very little, if any, corrosion. This has been borne out by the fact that many amalgam fillings will last for twenty years or more. However, recent research shows that mercury *does* leak out of the filling, and that corrosion occurs more rapidly in the presence of acidic drinks, hot food, sugar and strong chemicals. Most importantly, there is also corrosion from bacteria where the oral hygiene is poor. There is much dispute over how much mercury is released, and the debate centres around the question, 'Are these micro-quantities harmful?'

Mercury toxicity. Mercury is found in many of the foods we eat and can be present in the air and water. There is no doubt that the skeletons of modern man contain higher levels of mercury than our ancestors of even several hundred years ago. The cause of this increase is not due primarily to our fillings, but to mercury used in the fungicides and industrial wastes which pollute our seas and rivers.

Some forms of mercury such as methyl-mercury are very toxic, and there have been two notable examples of mass poisonings. In Minimata Bay in Japan in 1953, polluted tuna fish were eaten and some forty-six people died. The fish were contaminated by an industrial discharge containing mercurial catalysts used in the manufacture of plastics. The Iraq disaster of 1972, following on from previous mercury poisonings involving fatalities, was by far the worst. Over 450 people died and over 6,000 were admitted to hospital after eating bread made from seed which had been treated with a methyl-mercury fungicide. Because of these disasters, however, scientists were given the opportunity to study in detail the effects of mercury on the body. Methyl-mercury is fat-soluble, can be quickly absorbed by the body, and concentrates in the nervous system and the kidneys. All parts of the body can be affected by this form of mercury poisoning, and symptoms can vary immensely from headaches and depression to numbness and death.

There are those who claim mercury as a fairly common cause of any undiagnosed complaints, and the list of symptoms is seemingly endless. As mercury toxicity can appear to mimic other diseases, I would argue that the other more common causative agents be considered before jumping to a diagnosis of mercury toxicity.

Is there a way of knowing whether a patient is suffering from mercury toxicity? The answer appears to be inconclusive. As with any other disease or malfunction of the body, a full and detailed medical and psychological history may provide some valuable clues, for all good diagnosticians are detectives at heart! In other countries such as the USA, some dentists are now providing a diagnostic service for amalgam toxicity. The type of investigations they provide may be as follows:

1 An initial screening which consists of:
   a) Clinical examination
   b) Mercury sensitivity patch test
   c) Intraoral galvanic current measurement
2 A bio-electronic evaluation
3 A comprehensive evaluation which includes:
   a) Complete blood count
   b) Blood serum profile
   c) Mercury blood level
   d) Mercury urine level
   e) Electrocardiogram
   f) Intraoral mercury vapour measurement.

There may often be a divergence of opinion regarding the results of the above investigations. It is also true that some practitioners use alternative methods of diagnosis such as acupuncture, electro-diagnosis, homoeopathy and kinesiology (see Chapter Eleven). This is where there may be some conflict with the more conventional diagnosticians.

But someone who firmly believes she suffered from mercury toxicity is a British ex-nurse, Helen Roper. Three years previously, she had become ill for no apparent reason, and was confined to a wheelchair feeling unnaturally tired and depressed. After having little success with conventional therapy, she attended a clinic in Nevada, where a diagnosis was made using a combination of the above-mentioned techniques, and in association with the fact that there had been a recent dental filling using amalgam. She was instructed to have all her mercury fillings replaced, and she took a course of tablets to remove mercury from her body. Within a few months she started to recover her health, and is now happy, healthy and active. This is not an isolated case, and I am keeping an open mind on this subject.

White patches in the mouth. During a recent international symposium, Professor Söremark, a dental consultant from Sweden, commented upon a condition called lichen planus. Patients who have this condition often show white patches or striations on the mucous membranes of the mouth, often the cheek tissue. Other areas of the body can be affected, and can be both painful and distressing. It is generally believed this condition is brought about by stress. Professor Söremark surprised many by claiming that when all the mercury fillings were removed and a detoxification programme was administered to remove mercury from the body, *every one* of his patients was cured. For all the symptoms of lichen planus to disappear may take up to a year following this programme, but when questioned about such an astonishing cure rate, he said that similar results have been achieved in other hospitals in Sweden and Norway.

Threat to the unborn? During pregnancy, expectant mothers are advised to visit their dentist. This is quite correct, especially from a holistic viewpoint, as explained previously. This is also the time when treatment carried out through the general dental services is free. However, it is *not* the time to have treatment involving amalgam fillings unless strictly necessary. It has been shown that mercury can cross the placental membrane and actually concentrate in the foetus. Breast milk may also contain high levels of mercury. Research results indicate that when an existing mercury filling is removed from a tooth or a new amalgam is placed in a cavity, there is an increase in mercury vapour which can be inhaled. The methods used in dentistry today such as high-velocity suction and liberal quantities of water used to cool the tip of the drill minimize the amount of mercury vapour to which the patient is exposed. However, just as dentists are very conscientious about not giving their pregnant patients X-rays, no matter how small the radiation dose, I feel the same should apply to treatment involving amalgam fillings. After all, if there are a few 'leaky' or cracked fillings, a wait until after lactation should not lead to any serious problems, especially if diet and oral hygiene are good. Treatment will still be free for up to one year after the baby is born.

Remember, after conception, do *not* have fillings replaced

unnecessarily even for other non-mercury fillings, and do not be concerned about your existing mercury fillings. The potential release of mercury vapour from these will be microscopic.

Electricity in the mouth. The mouth is a very active place electrically as well as chemically. Whenever different metals are present in a solution or, in this case, saliva, little 'batteries' can be formed. Many people notice this effect: if a metal filling is touched by a fork, or when a piece of silver paper is inadvertently chewed, the reaction is often a sharp jolt of pain. This represents an electric current forming in the mouth and teeth, activating the nerves that register sensation.

Dentists use a range of metals and their alloys, and amalgam, crowns and dentures can be constructed from gold, silver, chromium, cobalt, stainless steel etc. As it is common to have several of these present in the mouth simultaneously, there is no doubt that electric currents and therefore electro-magnetic fields can be produced. One has only to place a micro-volt meter on different teeth in the mouth, especially those containing fillings or crowns, to vividly illustrate the wide range of electrical potentials. Some practitioners use a sophisticated form of volt meter as an indicator for suspected reactions to mercury fillings, but this is not a conclusive test.

There is, however, a much broader question. The communication network of the nervous system works by the generation of electrical impulses. As the mouth geographically sits next to the brain and the main trunk of nerves that radiate from the brain to the rest of the body, what effect could these electrical disturbances in the mouth be having on the messages received by the rest of the body? Could they be affecting our general health? Many researchers, especially those working in acupuncture and radionics, are concerned (see Chapter Eleven). I personally feel that this is a fascinating area for new research, and present biophysical investigations may have far-reaching ramifications.

Mercury: the added burden. It is argued by many concerned with environmental medicine that man today is plagued by many pollutants, especially in food. Together these pollutants increase the body burden — how hard our bodies are required to work to maintain health. Every added burden increases the risk of disease. Many believe that mercury, even in small amounts, may just tip the balance in favour of disease. Mercury may not be the sole causative agent, but could be 'the straw that breaks the camel's back'. If this is the case then, unfortunately, we are likely to see an increase in the number of cases where the disease or malfunction may have been triggered by mercury, as there appears to be little sign of other environmental pollutants diminishing. This is placing mercury toxicity in a much broader context. By eating and living in a healthier environment, I am sure that mercury would play an even smaller role in affecting our health, not least because, through good diet, we would require fewer fillings.

COMPOSITES

These normally describe the tooth-coloured materials, which, until recently, have been used on the front teeth only. For it is still generally considered that composite fillings are not so durable, and will require replacement at more frequent intervals than amalgam fillings – every five to ten years, say. But the quality is constantly being improved from the point of view of cosmetics, strength and longevity, and due to recent improvements in their strength, for instance, they can now be placed in back teeth where the chewing pressures and stresses are greatest. These are proving successful, and are now seen as a viable alternative to amalgam – and of course they look much nicer.

They are composed of a mixture of a very advanced form of acrylic (plastic) and a filler. This can be very finely ground quartz (glass) or silica (sand), to put it crudely. Mixed together their combined properties can give extremely tooth-like characteristics: for instance, when light shines through these materials, the pattern of colours can imitate exactly the natural shades and translucencies seen in a tooth. At present there are two systems of setting the composite material: one is to mix two pastes thoroughly together – similar to some strong glues! – and the other set is obtained by shining either an ultra-violet or strong white light on to the filling newly placed in the tooth. The latter is particularly useful when fillings are more complicated or when cosmetic work requires a longer construction time.

Many people now believe that they would be happier if their

mercury fillings were replaced by composite. Apart from the undoubted cost of this replacement in terms of actual cash and of dental time, there is the consideration that none of the effects of *these* materials have been fully investigated. For it is conceivable that people may have allergic reactions to the constituents of composites, just as they might to mercury. I feel this is unlikely, however, in the majority of cases.

GOLD

Gold is perhaps the oldest of dental materials, and is arguably still one of the best. It is very strong, hard-wearing, non-toxic and very compatible with the tooth. It has disadvantages, though, and to many the main one is cosmetic. We north Europeans tend to favour the 'natural' look, whereas our Mediterranean cousins often prefer to display their wealth in their teeth! Cost, too, of course, plays an important part in the choice of gold for fillings, for it is undoubtedly more expensive, and it also requires more clinical time in its preparation and fitting.

Crowns

Crowning – or 'capping' as it's popularly known – is normally carried out when teeth have been heavily filled and are either very unsightly or extremely weak. There are two main sorts of crowns. A jacket crown fits like a cap after the dentist has reduced the size of the underlying tooth by drilling it, rather like giving it a 'short back and sides'. Thereafter it will have a peg-like shape. A post crown is used when a tooth is dead and has been root filled, and may have discoloured and become brittle. The part of the tooth above the gumline normally used to secure the crown will not be strong enough. A post is therefore placed into the root and a crown can then be fixed to the post – usually constructed in gold, but can be made in other materials, such as stainless steel. If crowns are prepared and fitted properly, then they will last for many, many years. Because they fit completely over the tooth and should fit very tightly, there should certainly not be any tooth decay. By regular careful brushing around the gumline where the crown fits the tooth, and with the use of dental floss, crowns should be trouble-free and cosmetically very pleasing. In my opinion, crowned teeth are much less liable to be attacked by tooth decay than natural ones.

Most crowns today are constructed in a dental laboratory. The dentist will take accurate impressions of the teeth in the mouth, and these will enable the dental technician to design and construct a crown that will complement the existing dentition. The materials the technician can use are various.

PORCELAIN

This was the most favoured for front teeth because, cosmetically, it looks very natural. However, as with porcelain china, it can be brittle, and where the crown is under extreme pressure, breakages can and do occur.

BONDED PORCELAIN

When strength is required as well as a good cosmetic look, porcelain is thermo-chemically bonded to an underlying base of gold or other metal alloy. The metal will normally be completely covered by the porcelain, and, although this method may once have meant a dull-looking tooth, good technicians these days can achieve near perfect results.

Bonded crowns can be used to restore back or molar teeth, and this usage is becoming more popular, especially with those patients who would like to present the image of a filling-free mouth.

GOLD

Where cosmetics may not be a major consideration – on the back teeth, say – a large proportion of crowns are made from gold. This can be of a high percentage gold, giving a yellow coloration, or an alloy, which will give a shiny silvery appearance. These are immensely strong and, in many cases, are infinitely preferable to an extraction.

Due to the inherent properties of gold, the crowns constructed of gold need not fit entirely over the whole tooth: in some circumstances, an inlay – or a three-quarter crown – may be considered more appropriate.

Replacing Missing Teeth

It still amazes me that so many people nowadays walk around quite unashamedly with unsightly gaps because of missing teeth. Besides the social and speech implications of this, it may also mean that the patient has problems of inefficient mastication and thus of digestion. A vast majority of adults do, in fact, have sufficient missing teeth to create gaps and, in theory, these ought to be filled by some form of dental appliance, usually a bridge or a denture or a combination of both.

BRIDGEWORK

It is generally accepted that, where it is practicable, bridgework represents the most successful way of filling a gap. From the wearer's point of view, bridges are comfortable, stable and cosmetically pleasing. Because they occupy no more than the area of the missing tooth or teeth, patients quickly become used to them, often commenting that the bridges are like a natural part of their mouth. Most bridges are firmly fixed to supporting teeth, and so the fear that they might fall out at an inopportune moment is immediately diminished! And, as most bridges are constructed using bonded porcelain, they are as natural looking as the bonded crowns already mentioned.

Bridges are so-called because that is exactly what they are doing – they are bridging a gap just as a bridge spans a river or ravine. And similar engineering principles have to be utilized if long-term success is to be achieved. The support structures for bridgework are often the adjacent teeth, and they need to be sound and strong in their foundation as they are obviously being asked to carry a greater load. As with crowning, much of the design and construction is carried out in the dental laboratory. This requires a great deal of skill and precision from both dentist and technician.

Types of bridges. The most common, and arguably the most secure, type of bridge is that in which the replacement tooth or teeth is/are suspended between the adjacent teeth. This tooth, made of bonded porcelain normally, is attached to its supporting pillars which are often crowned or part crowned as a basic of the bridge structure. Occasionally, the replacement tooth is attached to the support on one side only, and this is known as a cantilever system. The permutations on these basic principles are many, and the dentist will match his skills to the individual problems as they present themselves.

A very recent innovation is that of the bonded bridge. This represents a breakthrough in both technology and conservative dentistry. If the teeth adjacent to a missing tooth have not been filled or damaged to any great extent, it would be a shame to reduce them for crowning, and the bonded bridge is an ideal solution. The back surface enamel of the sound teeth is 'conditioned', lightly etched with a very mild acid, which microscopically roughens the surface; thereafter allowing composite material to stick the bridge firmly in position by means of unseen metal tags. Again, the missing tooth can be constructed of a bonded porcelain.

Precision attachments. These are used when the gap to be spanned is too large or unsuitable for a bridge to be successful. The principles of design are partly that of bridgework and partly that of dentures. They are similar to a bridge in that they just span the space between teeth and utilize the adjacent teeth for their support and retention. They are similar to a denture, however, as some of the support is derived from the underlying gum, and they can be removed for cleaning.

PARTIAL DENTURES

There are circumstances when, because of the situation in the mouth, or because of cost, the use of bridgework is not feasible. Although people regard dentures with a certain distaste, they *can* be designed so that they are comfortable, unobtrusive and secure.

Types of partial dentures. There are two main types: acrylic based and metal based. The main advantages of acrylic dentures are that they are relatively inexpensive and easier to design and construct. They are held in position by a combination of snug fit between the teeth and an adhesion of the plastic base of the denture and the salivary moisture on the gum. Sometimes additional clips are used. Although they are usually well tolerated, there are many potential problems in that they can predispose to gum disease unless very carefully designed, are often bulky in the mouth, and, if someone has a strong bite, they are prone to breakage.

Dentures of metal, the most popular material employed, are an alloy of chrome and cobalt. Although the thought of a metal denture conjures up a vision of Jaws in some of the James Bond films, they can be made unobtrusive, lightweight and secure. Chrome-cobalt dentures require a great deal of design precision and care, because, for their retention, they utilize the existing teeth as well as the gums, and, as they are designed to both clasp and rest on the natural teeth, there is far less movement. The metal base can be of a very fine construction covering very little of the surface of the mouth. This gives metal dentures an obvious advantage over acrylic as bacteria are much less likely to accumulate under the plate, and the denture will feel less obtrusive to the patient. A surprising aspect is that, in comparison to acrylic, the metal feels very much more natural to many patients.

Cosmetic Dentistry

Gleaming white teeth are intimately associated with beauty and good health. If you are happy with your teeth – just as you might be with a hairstyle, say – you will be happy in yourself and reflect an inner confidence. From another viewpoint, a disfigured smile due to gaps or staining will create an adverse impression, however well presented the owner might be in every other way. If you are unhappy with the appearance of your teeth, it is likely that you will pay less attention to them, and this could lead to further problems. Cosmetic dentistry therefore can play an important part in any holistic dentist's approach. For it has often been observed that, by restoring a patient's pride in his appearance through cosmetic work, the patient can also revitalize an interest in every other aspect of his appearance, and of his health. In many cases, it can even involve a happy change of personality – and indeed quality of life.

CROWN AND BRIDGEWORK

The perfect teeth we admire in film stars and pop stars are very probably the product of expensive cosmetic crown and bridge-work! For not only can crowns and bridges improve the appearance by filling gaps, they can also change the shape, size and colour of teeth that may be misaligned, heavily filled, or stained. This type of treatment is not necessarily only available to the very wealthy, as most high-street practitioners have sufficient skill and expertise to provide a similar service.

FILLINGS AND VENEERS

Crowns and bridgework are normally rather expensive, but to improve the appearance considerably may require only subtle changes to the existing teeth. Discoloured fillings can be replaced with composites, and discoloured teeth and unsightly stains can be treated by a veneer technique. This literally is the application of a veneer, or thin composite layer, to a large discoloured area of the tooth; it adheres by means of the 'conditioning' or light acid etching already discussed. This technique can enable a whole tooth to radically change its appearance, both in colour and shape. The great advantage of this technique is that very little if any tooth needs to be drilled away, and the whole process can often be performed painlessly, without requiring any form of anaesthesia.

ORTHODONTICS

The general principles are discussed in Chapter Three, but ortho-dontics can certainly be regarded as the most effective form of cosmetic dentistry. It obviously requires, in the main, forward planning, and thus is of great relevance to our children. However, this does not mean that, in certain situations, adults may not benefit also from orthodontic procedures. The bones of an adult, of course, will be less flexible than a child's, so this may influence the length of time involved in producing effective movement of teeth. An orthodontic appliance is never very good-looking, but most adults will happily put up with a temporary disfigurement, motivated by the potential dental joys to come.

SURGICAL TREATMENT

Although rare, surgery can give immense cosmetic benefits. The most vivid example involves the congenital deformity of hare lip, where the bones and lip of the upper jaw have not grown together at birth. Today's cosmetic surgeons are so wonderfully skilled that, by the time the baby reaches adulthood, there is often little trace of this potentially most disfiguring condition.

Surgery can also dramatically improve the appearance of a grossly protruding lower jaw. Parts of the mandible are removed, and the chin can effectively be repositioned to give a more pleasing appearance.

Some Clinical Procedures

To achieve many of the above aims – with the exception perhaps of the veneers and orthodontics – much of dentistry involves uncomfortable if not painful procedures unless some form of pain avoidance is employed. And to achieve this painless state can often involve sensations which, to many, are distressing and inconvenient.

THE NEEDLE

Perhaps one of the most feared instruments the dentist possesses. Some areas of the mouth are more sensitive than others, but, if a good injection technique is used, the discomfort can be minimal. Today's needles, although mass produced, are extremely sharp, and after being used perhaps only once, are disposed of. This should obviate any fear of cross-contamination from such diseases as hepatitis and, more recently, AIDS. Dentists are made very much aware of the risks to themselves and to their patients, and all possible precautions are taken.

LOCAL ANAESTHESIA

Many dentists will often rub a small amount of anaesthetic paste in the area of the gum that is to receive the injection. This will even further minimize any painful pricking sensation.

There are various forms of local anaesthetic and the majority come in sterile sealed glass cartridges. One group have a chemical that restricts the blood supply to the area of the gum and which usually provides a longer period of numbness; another group of locals lack these properties, are still very effective, but have the advantage of causing fewer side effects. One of the chemicals used to restrict the blood supply is adrenalin; this occurs naturally in the body, but can interact with certain drugs such as anti-depressants. This is one reason why a dentist asks you if you are taking any medication as it may be relevant to the treatment he will give.

GENERAL ANAESTHESIA

Often, due to extreme fear or indeed phobia, certain people will not undertake any dental treatment unless they are unconscious. From a holistic point of view, I feel that this is a failing on the part of the dentist, and I believe that, in many cases, this situation can be altered by counselling and by techniques such as hypnosis (see below). There *is* a place for general anaesthesia – for difficult extractions, multiple extractions and for involved surgery of both jaws and gums – but I feel that it should never be undertaken without careful consideration. Although very rare, unfortunate incidents have occurred involving general anaesthesia, and today most dentists take the utmost care before, during and after administration.

RELATIVE ANALGESIA

A popular technique for the nervous patient is to give a combination of gas and air – nitrous oxide and oxygen – similar to that used during childbirth. This will bring on a state of relaxation and drowsiness without rendering the patient completely unconscious (and it is interesting to note that, in this relaxed condition, patients who are resistant to hypnosis will often succumb to suggestion).

Another method of inducing this relaxed state is by injecting a solution of Diazepam into the body via a vein. This technique has the advantage of producing a very profound loss of sensation, and it is also amnesic, in that the patient may often forget what has happened to him in the dentist's chair. However, Diazepam has side effects as do most drugs, so, from a holistic point of view, I would be happier to see a situation where such methods are not required.

HYPNOSIS

It is generally acknowledged that most people visit the dentist with a certain amount of trepidation, and even children who may be attending for the first time can be a little apprehensive of the man in the white coat. Any method of reducing this fear and making the time spent in the chair more comfortable is worth considering – and hypnosis may be the answer for many people.

At present the image of a hypnotist is distinctly dubious, with hints of a Rasputin-like power, and his skills are principally associated with the giving-up of habits such as smoking. However, many medical professionals have become aware of the potential of hypnosis and have undertaken postgraduate courses to both study and practise hypnotic techniques.

Although the art of hypnosis has been known for centuries, it was first recognized in a scientific sense when Anton Mesmer (from whom comes the word 'mesmerize') used it to cure psychosomatic conditions in the late eighteenth century. Dentists were using hypnosis in 1890 – as reported in the *BDJ* – in order to carry out extractions, and it was only with the advent of anaesthesia that the dental practice of hypnosis died out. Nearly 100 years later, hypnosis may have come full circle, and could be used in many aspects of dentistry, not least the relief of fear and pain.

The following is a brief list of some of the ways in which hypnosis can be of use to the patient and dentist.

1   Hypnosis can relax the patient, and this has the consequence of raising the pain threshold – the level at which one perceives pain.

2   Hypnosis can reduce phobias about things like needles, noise of the drill etc.

3   Hypnosis can be used to actually produce analgesia, to numb an area of the mouth to the extent that fillings – even extractions – can be carried out without the patient feeling any pain.

4   Many patients feel sick or want to gag when a dental instrument is put in the mouth or an impression is taken. Hypnosis can be used to eliminate this unwanted reflex.

5   There are several problems associated with orthodontic treatment, and one of these is the child not wanting to wear his or her brace. Hypnosis may be used to persuade them of the

error of their ways! Connected with orthodontics are the habits of thumb-sucking and nail-biting, which can have adverse effects of the shape of the jaw. Hypnosis can also be used to stop these.

6 Most trained hypnotists use a technique called ego strengthening. This is a method by which ideas and suggestions are given to the patient which will be to his benefit – and he can be made to feel calmer, more reassured and positive about himself and life in general.

7 A somewhat surprising finding, which is of great benefit to the dentist in particular, is that, under hypnosis, the patient appears to produce less saliva and, in the case of surgery, bleeds less and heals more rapidly. These phenomena appear to be associated with the autonomic nerve supply, and may have links with enhanced healing as described in Chapter Eleven.

There are as many hypnotic induction techniques as there are hypnotists, but I would like to make it perfectly clear that those in the medical and dental professions who use hypnosis are very responsible about any potential psychological problems. Remember that you cannot, under hypnosis, be forced to do anything you would not want to do, and it is not a devious technique for dentists to suggest you pay ten times the normal amount for treatment!

I believe hypnosis has a very exciting role to play in the futures of both medicine and dentistry, and it is encouraging to see ever-increasing numbers of doctors and dentists attending the training courses. Hypnotic suggestion is, of course, practised routinely by many a dentist. By a kind and caring approach, there is a greater likelihood that you will have faith in what he tells you. If it is suggested to you that the introduction of the needle will be a mere tickle, then this is usually all that your brain will perceive.

X-RAYS

These are a very important diagnostic tool for the dentist, and I would go so far as to say that, in certain situations, they are invaluable. With a difficult impacted wisdom tooth, for instance, the position of the tooth in relation to the surrounding bone and nerves can, if not forewarned by an X-ray, cause serious surgical complications. One survey found that, on routine scanning of the teeth and jaws by X-ray, some 40 per cent extra pathologies came to light. These included bone cysts, buried teeth and roots, and abscesses.

Most X-rays taken at the dentist involve the use of a small piece of film that is placed in the mouth, and the exposure of the patient is minimal. Larger external scan X-rays (OPGs), are also popular, especially when considering oral surgery and orthodontics.

The dental profession are very conscientious about the hazards of X-rays, and recent legislation has ensured that even stricter controls on both equipment and usage have been instituted. However, from a holistic viewpoint, I would like to see X-rays used only when it is considered completely necessary.

CHAPTER TEN

Holistic Dentistry

A well-known speaker at a recent dental conference divided dentists into three categories: teeth dentists, mouth dentists and whole person dentists. I strive to be a whole person, or holistic, dentist. I believe that every reaction in the mouth affects the whole body, and that reactions in the body have a profound influence in the mouth. After all, the blood that runs to our mouths is the same blood that runs to our toes, and the bone which supports the teeth consists of exactly the same materials as the bones upon which we stand. By following this philosophy, the holistic dentist is not just concerned with treating the *effects* of disease, but is looking for the fundamental *cause*. It is generally recognized that the common cold is brought on by a virus; however, a holistic view would be that the basic cause is the inability of the body to fight off that virus.

Nutrition and Stress

I firmly believe that nutrition is the cornerstone of dental health and that, were we able to have a 'perfect' diet, the vast majority of treatments would not be necessary. This is a somewhat bold statement, and could be criticized in most professional spheres, both medical and dental. Most diseases, of course, are multi-factorial, and indeed there is a vast individual variation but, if the diet is totally compatible with an individual, then the disease process could be eliminated. This in scientific terms is regarded as ortho-molecular nutrition, which basically is a sophisticated way of saying that if a growing body is given all its nutrients in the right proportions, it will then grow to its fullest potential. Similarly, the chromosomes of the genetic structure, fed on the ideal diet, will then duplicate as nature intended them to. Given the ideal diet, the adult will be able to repair and maintain all the tissues of the body. This is the general principle by which most nutritionists work, and as it is relevant to the health of the body in general, so it is to the health of the jaws and teeth.

THE STATE OF THE NATION

In any conversation, it doesn't take long before the subject of health crops up, and in fact, this is the very first greeting most people receive: 'How are you?' Very often this can lead into a blow-by-blow account of the latest malady, be it major or minor. If a visitor from outer space were to examine the vast majority of people living in the UK, he would have to conclude that we were a nation of health cripples. In fact, one commentator has suggested that we are standing 'on the very edge of the abyss of a crisis of epidemic magnitude, such as the world has never known before, including chronic poisoning, heart and artery disease, cerebral strokes, diseases of the nervous system, mental and emotional disorders, rampant dental decay, congenital malformations and degenerative conditions of all sorts' (*Nutrition Science and Health Education*, Dr C. Curtis Shears). If you don't believe me, then how does 300 million working days lost with certified illness sound? This cost the country in excess of 2,000 million pounds, and all in one year! Is the cost of the National Health Service diminishing? The answer is a categorical no, and we are still short of medical staff, equipment, and facilities, and the future looks rather bleak.

THE FOUR STRESSES

Many believe that the majority of disease in the west is primarily caused by our so-called civilized society. This lifestyle is inextricably linked with stress. Many healers will often break this stress down into a number of categories, although all are interdependent. The major stresses may be defined as environmental, emotional, physical and nutritional, not necessarily in that order.

A certain amount of stress is good for us, and acts in some cases as a form of motivation. But it is the level of stress that is important: too much will lead to disease.

Environmental. This is the one over which the average person has no control, although environmental groups are beginning to make their voices heard. It's not only the eccentrics in their smocks and sandals who are demanding change, but well-respected scientists, physicians, and many well-educated people from all walks of life. What we as a society are doing to our global environment has already directly affected individual health – think of the mercury poisonings in Japan and Iraq. It is universally agreed that if many of the directives below were followed, our environment would be dramatically improved.

1 Reduce industrial effluents. Look how the fish life in the Thames has proliferated since anti-pollution measures were taken. Think about the smogs of London caused by the unchecked churning out of fumes from factory chimneys. And how the Norwegians are protesting about the acid rain polluting their forests and rivers – a rain which is thought to originate in the British Isles.

2 Phase out long-acting chemical pesticides and herbicides. Science should be used to develop natural and organic alternatives which are bio-degradable. For, with the use of chemicals such as DDT, whole populations of birds of prey were annihilated. What effect might this have had on our bodies?

3 Recycle industrial and domestic wastes. This has obvious advantages in that it will not drain the earth of further valuable resources, and this is, to a limited extent, already carried out with glass and paper. The composting of waste food will return valuable trace elements to the soil.

4 Reduce the use of petro-chemicals. A lot is known about the deleterious effects of car exhaust fumes, but much less is known about the harm that could be caused by petro-chemical products in food, water, air, pesticides, cosmetics, detergents and drugs.

Emotional. It is well known, both inside the medical profession and out, that the state of the mind plays a major role in the general health and well-being of the body. After the death of a spouse, it is not uncommon for the surviving partner also to die within a fairly short space of time, or to develop a very serious illness of some sort, especially if the love bond between them has been strong. Conversely, a patient who has been pronounced incurable can often have a remission entirely through determination and strength of will.

These are vivid illustrations, but we all suffer from less significant, but none the less important, day-to-day emotional stresses. Executives may regard their jobs as the most stressful, but worry over how to manage the housekeeping or about an examination can create similar levels of stress in other individuals. We all react to stress in different ways and every situation will elicit varying responses from differing individuals. However, psychiatrists and researchers have drawn up a scale to help them measure life stress and find out how much stress piles up before illness sets in. 'The Social Adjustment Rating Scale' (as taken from an article in the *Journal of Psychosomatic Research* by T. H. Holmes and R. H. Rahe) covers over forty significant life events which are graded from 100 down to 11 (the last being a parking ticket). We reproduce the top 15.

Life Event	
1 Death of spouse	100
2 Divorce	73
3 Marital separation from spouse	65
4 Detention in jail or other institution	63
5 Death of a close family member	63
6 Major personal injury or illness	53
7 Marriage	50
8 Being fired at work	47
9 Marital reconciliation with mate	45
10 Retirement from work	45
11 Major change in the health or behaviour of a family member	44
12 Pregnancy	40
13 Sexual difficulties	39
14 Gaining a new family member (through birth, adoption, relative moving in)	39
15 Major business readjustment (merger, reorganization, bankruptcy etc.)	39

Physical. There is a greater awareness these days of the need to keep in shape, and there has been an unprecedented boom in gymnasia, slimming clinics and health farms, and in participant sports, especially those requiring a lot of physical activity. Many more now believe in the old adage, *mens sana in corpore sano*, a healthy mind in a healthy body.

In times of danger, our ancestors produced hormones in their bodies which would better prepare them to either stand and fight or turn and flee. These hormones speeded up the heart beat, increased blood pressure, tensed the muscles and quickened the breathing. All very useful when facing that sabre-toothed tiger, but not so relevant when worrying about how to pay the gas bill, for today's stresses call forth the same hormones. If these induced tensions are not relieved, they are inclined to build up and cause stress. Physical exercise is one of the best ways of reducing tensions, and competitive sports are also useful in relieving aggression.

Posture, or the lack of it, can also contribute to physical stress on the body. If we sit, stand or lie incorrectly, the bone structure and associated muscles are not in balance. These imbalances can lead to pain, discomfort and degeneration. Many new sciences are evolving to combat and treat disease which derive from these postural stresses, like osteopathy, chiropractic and kinesiology (see Chapter Eleven).

Dietary. We are what we eat, and if you think about it, we can be nothing else. After all, what else are we made of but what we consume and what we breathe. If we feed ourselves with rubbish, the result is obvious.

The body digests food through a long and complicated process which begins, as we know, in the mouth: if that food is of poor quality – over-refined, contaminated, laden with additives – and is in incorrect proportions for the body's requirements, there can be internal stresses. The whole digestive and metabolic system has to work harder to properly process the nutrients that the body needs.

It is often considered that we in the west do not suffer from malnutrition. However, vitamin and mineral deficiencies and their related diseases are becoming increasingly commonplace, and these, surprisingly, are often caused by *over-* rather than by *under-*eating. It is the over-consumption of empty calories –

found in refined sugar and carbohydrates – and the over-consumption of protein and fat which give rise to the majority of the illnesses that fill our hospitals and dental chairs. Perhaps we ought to take the advice of the 'Father of Medicine', for Hippocrates wrote in 460 BC, 'Foods must be in the condition in which they are found in nature, or at least, in a condition as close as possible to that found in nature. Let your food be your medicine and your medicine your food.'

Stress and disease. There is a concept that if a person exceeds a certain stress threshold then disease will result. Imagine a stress threshold of 100. If we give points for the above mentioned stresses then they all have a cumulative effect on one's health or lack of it: the higher the figure the nearer to disease we come and vice versa. Let's give an example. Mr X's diet is poor which could count for some 35 points; he lives in the centre of the city which adds on another 30, say; his job is sedentary but he exercises twice a week, which adds 15 points; and has a happy marriage and steady job which means another 10. His total count is below the theoretical disease level, but if he moves house – a well-known stress factor, say of 20 – Mr X could complain of depression, headaches, back pain and indigestion.

By lowering any or all of the contributory stresses, his health could be restored, although some would be very difficult to alter. Diet, however, can be simple to modify, and can often bring beneficial results in a very short space of time. The ideal situation, therefore, is obviously one in which the levels of stress attached to each area of life are low, and we should all strive to this end.

The dentist may observe when stress is reaching a high level. For he is in a unique position as he will often be examining his patients at regular intervals which will be long enough apart for noticeable changes to occur. Orally, the manifestations can be an increase in gum disease, excessive wear on the teeth due to night-grinding, and patients complaining of such things as dryness in the mouth and bad breath. By further questioning and more detailed examination, perhaps of the whole body, disease in its early stages may be diagnosed and, where necessary, referred to the appropriate healer. The dentist could now be taking a new role in society by acting as an early-warning health screen, and could become involved in more direct health care such as nutritional programmes.

Holistic Examinations

During their long training, dentists study many aspects of medicine which are very necessary to dental practice. Seemingly irrelevant medical information may have a profound influence on how the dentist interprets dental problems, and will influence the treatment thereafter. Thus every dentist is, in a sense, holistic, in that he will be considering more than just the mouth, especially when undertaking the initial verbal examination.

THE MEDICAL HISTORY

For this reason, when you visit a dentist for the first time, you are confronted with a barrage of questions. Many of these questions involve your past medical history, and although they could occasionally seem to be a little too personal for the man who's supposed to be filling your teeth, he is asking them for very specific reasons. It may seem particularly impertinent when a dentist asks a single female patient if she is on the pill: as we have already seen, this is extraordinarily relevant to a gum problem. If the dentist asks whether a patient has had rheumatic fever, it is because there is a unique relationship – potentially fatal – between the consequences of the disease and dental treatment.

Rheumatic fever, which would normally be diagnosed by a doctor, occurs most commonly in childhood. It can start with a sore throat, make the joints and limbs very painful and swollen, and the kidneys can also be affected. It's not likely that you would be unaware of having this disease as it can cause considerable distress for as long as eight weeks.

However, a major consequence of rheumatic fever may be damage to the lining and the valves of the heart. Should certain bacteria which live in the mouth escape into the bloodstream and gain access to these areas of damaged tissue in the heart, a very serious infection can ensue (sub-acute bacterial endocarditis).

This can lead, if untreated, to heart failure and death. Dental treatment as routine as a scaling, and certainly a dental extraction, can give rise to this bacterial release. People who have a history of rheumatic fever may also have a heart murmur, although this is not always the case. It is vital for anyone who has had rheumatic fever to maintain scrupulous mouth hygiene, and it is vital that they inform their dentist. The very same principles apply to any person who has had heart surgery, especially that involving valve replacement.

Questions about your liver or whether you have ever been jaundiced are relevant to transmittable viral diseases such as hepatitis. This disease is highly contagious via the blood, and although fully recovered, the sufferer may still be a carrier for many years afterwards. The dentist will need to know this so that he can take all the appropriate safeguards.

The barrage may continue with questions on whether you are taking any medications, drugs, whether you smoke, drink to excess, have any allergies, have had any major operations or neurological symptoms. In fact, virtually everything that a doctor would need to know for a thorough insurance medical.

Very few dentists, however, will ask whether you suffer from migraines or frequent headaches, or from chronic pain in your back, and other parts of the body. A holistic dentist will find significance in the answers you give for it could be that these symptoms may relate to a jaw condition known as the TMJ syndrome (see page 186). At this stage, the questions may even elicit information about past involvement in car accidents etc., and any stresses to which you might have been subjected.

THE DENTAL HISTORY

After the medical questions will come the dental questions. A priority question should always be 'Do your gums bleed?', and we all know the ramifications of that. For new patients it is very relevant for the dentist to know the last time you had any treatment, as this will indicate the rate of progress of any dental disease, especially the accumulation of dental calculus. Pain is another major consideration, of course, but the dentist will want you to be very specific about its nature: where, type, intensity, frequency, duration and its stimulus. From this verbal interrogation alone, much can be gleaned about the condition of your teeth and gums.

The holistic dentist will also be interested to know about clicking and creaking noises on opening and closing the mouth; if you grind your teeth; frequent sinusitis; dizziness; ringing or popping in the ears; and if you experience a feeling that your teeth don't meet properly. If the answers to any of the above are affirmative, this could also indicate jaw dysfunction. Questions that might also have nutritional significance may be asked, such as frequent ulcers, sore tongue, cold sores and frequent cracks at the corners of the mouth.

PHYSICAL IMPRESSIONS

First impressions count. Those initial summings-up are often subconscious, but the holistic dentist will deliberately include them in his examination and may well make copious notes to that effect. How many people notice, and realize the significance of, say, things like a crooked smile, a nose that slopes to one side of the face, or one eye which does not open as much as the other? How many people are conscious of one shoulder lower than the other (likewise with the breasts), one leg longer than the other, or an incorrectly postured head? The holistic dentist regards all these seemingly minor aberrations with professional interest, for once again they could be signs of skeletal imbalance which in turn may affect the jaw.

As soon as you sit in the dental chair, he will be able to observe the colour of your complexion, the texture of your hair and skin, the condition of your eyes, any rashes or spots, or irregular swellings on either face or neck. Ruddy cheeks could suggest very high blood pressure; lank hair could mean a recent illness (a hairdresser would come to the same conclusion); protruding eyes may indicate an over-active thyroid; rashes or spots could indicate either hormonal imbalances, allergies or mineral and vitamin deficiencies. Nails, too, could show the latter, suggesting certain types of anaemia or serious zinc shortage. These are all simply indications, and I am sure no dentist, or doctor for that matter, would immediately rush to a firm diagnosis.

Before looking in your mouth, the dentist may want to feel your neck and jaw muscles to see if there are any irregularities – swollen glands, say, or inflammation in the tissues surrounding the mouth. Do not be alarmed if he sticks a finger in either ear and shouts at you to open and close your mouth! He will be investigating the way in which the jaw mechanism is working.

OPEN WIDE, PLEASE

The big moment has arrived. Only now will the dentist look into your mouth, which is what you thought he would have done right at the beginning. Before actually examining the teeth, the dentist will have a good look around at all parts of the mouth – at the lips, cheek tissue, palate, tongue, the floor of the mouth, and as far back as the tonsils. Many of these have clinical significance.

The tongue, of course, has always been used as a classic indicator of health – think of the doctor asking you to stick your tongue out – and a number of symptoms can reveal themselves there. Vitamin B deficiency can make the tongue a deeper red in colour, and of a 'raw steak' appearance; heavy smoking or medical drug taking can give rise to a 'hairy' tongue which can look alarming, as the back of the tongue does literally have long strands growing from it (these can grow so long that they break off, but it is not a condition to worry about).

Oral cancer is very rare, but any white lesions or lumps and bumps in the floor of the mouth – especially underneath the tongue – need to be investigated. There are many other possible causes of swellings such as blocked salivary ducts, mumps, an enlarged lymph node, or even a chronic abscess from a tooth. If the blood vessels underneath the tongue are swollen or show signs of minute haemorrhage, this may indicate a Vitamin C deficiency, and this is particularly common in the elderly. An experienced practitioner can glean an enormous amount of information from this initial study of the mouth, not least from the texture, colour and the overall appearance of the tissues. As mentioned before, the interior of the mouth is very hardy and resilient, and does not readily succumb to infection or damage. This is borne out by the fact that the vast majority of the population have very little sign of disease in the soft tissues of the mouth.

It would be nice if we could say the same about the gums. Gum disease is nearly always painless, and, to the untrained eye, as we've said, even quite advanced disease may progress unnoticed.

To a dentist, however, even the mildest gum condition is immediately apparent. As his first priority is to care for the foundation of the teeth, he will look very carefully at the gums, often using a special probe to measure the depth of the gum pockets.

Oddly enough, the teeth are examined last of all. The dentist will be looking for dental cavities, at the condition of existing fillings and crowns, and at the relationship between the individual teeth. He will look for other signs such as excessive wear (due to over-enthusiastic brushing, perhaps), abrasion on the biting surfaces (which may indicate grinding), and at how the top and bottom teeth come together. Erosion or the chemical wearing away of the teeth – possibly caused by too high a citrus fruit and drink intake – can be spotted at this stage as well. By virtue of his very intense light, the dentist can easily see many of the above, and indeed because the teeth are, to a certain extent, translucent, he can often detect the earliest signs of tooth decay which may not be picked up by the dental probe.

The relationship between the teeth and gums is, of course, what the dentist is primarily interested in, because there lie the origins of dental disease. As previously discussed, the shape, the position, the crowding and the function are all contributory factors, and at this time the dentist will be able to assess the effect these may have singularly or plurally on the condition of the patient's dental health. Poor hygiene will reveal itself now: it is often a source of amusement for many dentists when a child presents for examination with red and sore gums due to the unaccustomed extra brushing effort immediately beforehand. And the presence of large build-ups of calculus will reveal the areas of the mouth that are habitually brushed less efficiently.

Based on all these findings, the dentist will have a very clear picture, not just of the mouth but also of the general health and well-being of the patient. Further investigations may be required if the dentist feels they are necessary: he may take X-rays, take models of the teeth, refer the patient on to a dental specialist, recommend nutritional counselling or attendance at an osteopath, or indeed he may wish to liaise with the patient's general medical practitioner.

Holistic Treatments

The word 'holistic' means, in general terms, an involvement with the whole person. Many dentists, however, are reticent about allowing themselves to consider treating any other parts of the body except the head and neck. Their training concentrated on the anatomy, physiology, biochemistry and disease of everything above the shoulders, and correctly so as, after all, they wanted to be specialists in the mouth. But it is becoming increasingly apparent that dentists will have to look beyond those boundaries if they want to play a greater role in the treatment of their patients.

THE TMJ SYNDROME

A substantial proportion of the population suffer from migraines or frequent headaches. Over a third of these may have their origins in skeletal imbalance and malfunction of the joints that connect the lower jaw to the skull, just below the ears. These are called the tempero-mandibular joints (TMJ). That problems can occur here will be more easily understood if one considers that the lower jaw – the mandible – is the only moving bone that functions on *both sides of the body*. When these joints do not work in unison, then malfunction will follow, giving rise to an extraordinary list of symptoms. Although the TMJ syndrome has been recognized for many years, it is only recently that the far-reaching bodily consequences have been appreciated. And this is a classic example of where a holistic approach will pay handsome dividends in the understanding and treating of this common condition.

For common it is, and many headaches, migraines, back and neck pains, dizzy spells and ailments like chronic sinusitis, sore throats, tension and insomnia can be the direct result of the TMJ syndrome. Many osteopaths, for instance, have recognized that much back pain stems from a jaw dysfunction, and until recently, there has been very little clinical exchange between them and the dental profession. And there are many TMJ syndrome sufferers who are taking pain-killers, muscle relaxants and anti-depressants because their symptoms have not been properly diagnosed. This may all sound unlikely, and of course all the above mentioned have other medical origins, but a good TMJ specialist should be able to reach an accurate diagnosis by a summation of the relevant signs and symptoms.

The head weighs generally between 4 and 6 kg (9–14 lb), and balances on the end of a very flexible pole, the spine. That balance is maintained by the muscles of the shoulders, neck and lower jaw. When the latter is not balanced properly, the head can be thrown off true and the supporting muscles will have to strain to keep it in its proper position on the neck. This can result in muscle strain and asymmetries throughout the whole body, not just the face and neck, and this is what the holistic dentist would have looked out for during his first visual and physical examination of his patient.

If a TMJ syndrome is thought to be involved, muscles located as far apart as the temple and the calf of the leg may be palpated for signs of strain and tenderness. Don't suspect your dentist of less than professional motives, he is in pursuit of a clear diagnosis. X-rays of the jaw joints are also valuable, not just for establishing the way in which the lower jaw slots into its allotted place, but also to look for diseases such as arthritis. The position of the joints can also be assessed by the dentist placing his fingers in your ears! Try it for yourself: place a finger in either ear, press inwards and forwards, then open and close your mouth slowly. If you can feel the movement in the joint, and it is not the same on both sides, or there is clicking, then there may be a potential jaw dysfunction.

If there is a strong indication that the TMJs are involved, then the dentist will take models of your teeth. These will provide him with valuable information about how your teeth inter-relate, and will also provide the basis for making an appliance which, it is hoped, will relieve the symptoms. In the majority of cases, simply by fitting a plastic cover to either top or bottom teeth, this relief can be achieved. Why this is so is not fully understood, but it appears that by keeping the jaws in a non-habitual position, the muscles are given time to relax and rearrange themselves from their previously stressed position. The appliance will need to be worn continuously, especially during periods of uninterrupted concentration such as driving a car or writing a book(!), but especially during sleep.

There are some sufferers who, to obtain relief, require a much more accurate method of determining the correct relationship between their jaws. The types of appliance they require have to be carefully measured and constructed, and may initially feel completely alien, as if there were a brick in the mouth. There is rapid acceptance, however, when their symptoms and pain, as if by magic, completely disappear. Other health professionals may need to be brought in at this stage, including osteopaths, neurologists, doctors and physiotherapists, who may institute a programme of postural exercises.

Many people with lop-sided or malfunctioning jaw joints do not suffer any symptoms, but in a sense are walking 'time-bombs'. It is generally agreed that the TMJ syndrome is brought on by stress – whether dietary, emotional, environmental or physical – and if these stresses accumulate, and tilt the balance in favour of disease, they could trigger off the vast range of TMJ-related complaints. To both new sufferers, and all those who have experienced long-term pain, the knowledge and expertise of the dentist may offer hope.

Nutrition in Practice

'Dietary control of cavities and gum disease may soon replace the toothbrush and dental floss as the mainstay of a healthy mouth ... blood sample studies from more than 7,000 people and trace mineral analysis of their hair have led to the conclusion that dental disease is actually a whole body disease. . . . Tailoring diets to the needs of individual patients has produced remarkable results ... the diets worked for many patients unable to control dental disease with brushing and flossing.' These quotes, from an address to the Chicago Dental Society by Dr H. A. Huggins, encapsulate many of my own convictions, and confirm that in many other countries such as the USA, dentists have recognized the link between dietary control and dental health, and are prepared to be nutritional counsellors.

If you require advice on healthy eating in this country, to whom do you turn? At present, believe it or not, there are no universally recognized courses or diplomas in wholefood nutrition. There exists only a mish-mash of various food philosophies which, although they are all essentially related to each other, will give greater emphasis to one particular aspect of their subject. Most of this information can be gleaned from popular – and occasionally best-selling – books, but individual guidance is thin on the ground.

This is where there is a definite role for the natural or holistic dentist. Although doctors and dentists are not given any adequate dietary education at undergraduate level, their intimate knowledge of how the body works is essential for the deepest possible understanding and interpretation of nutritional principles. It is encouraging to see that many medical doctors are now utilizing these principles in their daily practice, and that a society devoted to nutritional medicine has recently been founded.

Most dentists do give some advice about nutrition, but usually no more than a discouragement of the use of sugar, and if this is ignored, they could well feel they would enjoy even less success when advocating a complete dietary change. The people who would most benefit from dental nutritional advice are those that are ill or are under stress, and both dentist and patient may become worried when disease processes in the mouth do not respond to treatment. For example, all dentists have seen patients who are meticulous in their oral hygiene, but who still suffer from degeneration of the oral tissues. If there are no other clinically significant factors to explain lack of healing response, this could in a sense be the motivation, and consequently a reappraisal of dietary habits may be undertaken and accepted more enthusiastically.

Every person is genetically and biochemically different, and the expression 'One man's meat is another man's poison' is a truism. Generalized dietary advice, no matter how sound the principles, may not be compatible with a particular individual, and so I feel nutritional counselling should only be undertaken on a one-to-one basis. It is essential to establish first of all the present nutritional status of the patient: this can be achieved by various means, but I find the most effective is a blood test. Through this we can not only look at the blood chemistry, but also at the blood cells and the circulating levels of minerals and vitamins. The blood chemistry will tell us the existing condition of many of the vital organs and glands through the amounts of chemicals like cholesterol, thyroid hormones, and albumin. There are many, and they all have individual and combined significance. The condition and number of the blood cells is obviously important, especially concerning things such as anaemia and chronic infections. But the levels of certain minerals and vitamins is, in some ways, what is most relevant to nutritional counselling.

The blood is not the only method, though, and analysis of hair, sweat, urine and faeces can be of great value in giving a complete nutritional picture. If properly undertaken, hair analysis has the unique advantage of being able to show the effects of nutrition over the several months of hair growth.

If two people eat exactly the same food, the amount of nutrients that each person will absorb and metabolize from that food will differ. The blood analysis will indicate what exactly is happening in the body, but the nutritionist will also want to know what food is being ingested to give these results. A diet sheet is one of the best ways of getting this information: the sheet, like the one reproduced opposite, will be filled in by the patient, listing everything he has eaten and drunk in a week (a shorter time wouldn't be appropriate). It is also important that the patient eats what he would normally consume during that week: a sudden guilty reliance on salads will not impress, and will not lead to any accurate conclusions.

After analysing both blood-test and diet-sheet results, the dentist may want to liaise with the patient's medical practitioner, especially if some of the findings require treatment the dentist is not qualified to carry out. If there are no basic medical problems, though, the dentist can make recommendations on any necessary dietary improvements. This will not necessarily just be supplementary vitamins and minerals, but could relate more to the balance and combination of foods: many, for instance, eat far too much protein and fat; others could be eating far too much fibre which is robbing them of essential minerals. From personal experience, I am often surprised by the results, but this only goes to confirm the vast biochemical individuality of each and every one of us.

The aim of the counselling will be to modify the patient's dietary habits, not only to make them healthier, but also to suit their lifestyle, social and economic status and, of course, their taste. To achieve these aims takes time, and it is wise for the counsellor to call the patient back after about six weeks to review

Diet Sheet

	Breakfast	Lunch	Dinner	Additional Snacks	Beverages e.g. Tea: Coffee: Alcohol
Monday					
Tuesday					
Wednesday					
Thursday					
Friday					
Saturday					
Sunday					

*Please enter *everything* you have eaten. Be completely honest with yourself. Remember this is to help and advise you to better health. Please enter brand names of foods where applicable.

progress. Some of the recommended dietary changes may not be suitable and further modifications may be required. Any extra minerals and vitamins that have been taken in this period must also be reviewed as I personally do not believe in long-term supplementation. Most of us, however, do seem to require an increase in our daily Vitamin C intake, and this, of course, is very important dentally.

Within as short a time as ten days, the patient can often see vast improvements in the condition in the mouth: the gums may have stopped bleeding, breath may be fresher, and the mouth feels generally 'cleaner'. In tandem with this, often go a new-found vitality, a fresher complexion, healthier hair and a sense of heightened well-being.

Dietary Guidelines from the Dentist

As with many things in life, one tends to set out with great enthusiasm and good intentions, but reality often intercedes and these resolutions soon weaken. I issue a series of simple advice sheets which I hope will strengthen my patients' resolve, and act as a memory jerker. These sheets also encompass many of the principles which I have been advocating throughout this book.

A WHOLEFOOD DIET

The term 'whole foods' is very simple, there is nothing cranky or off-putting about it. It simply means:

Foods which have nothing added or taken away.

Foods which are as near to their natural state as possible.

Foods which are not processed or refined.

Foods which do not contain artificial additives, flavourings, colours or preservatives.

Just 'whole' foods. It stands to reason that they must be better for you.

Sugar and salt. Forget them both!

Recent studies show that the daily salt or sodium requirement for a human being is probably no more than 200 milligrams a day.

This small quantity is available naturally in foods alone – in vegetables, meats and fish, fruits and grains – and no one should ever have to add salt to foods. The average amount taken in by most individuals is more than twenty-five times that amount. Salt seems to be at the root of hypertension, one of our most common twentieth-century illnesses. It also upsets the body's water balance. Once you start to omit salt from your cooking you will soon learn to do without it. Use fresh and dried herbs, garlic and spices for seasoning instead.

Refined sugar is a totally unnatural substance that has been stripped of any nutritional value. Sugar in concentrated form is very bad for the pancreas and consequently your energy levels. Also your teeth! Use honey and molasses to sweeten your food.

Fibre. This is an important factor in the diet, but if you eat a good wholefood diet you will be eating enough. Extra bran is not always beneficial. Wholemeal bread, plenty of salads and vegetables are the correct ways of providing nature's own filler.

Additives. Try to avoid whenever possible. These include colourings, preservatives and flavourings. Preservatives keep food 'larder' fresh long after it should have gone 'stale', a convenience for manufacturers. Colourings and flavourings are only needed because many people have come to expect them. If food needs disguising to make it taste good, wouldn't you do better without it?

Vitamins and minerals. Processing and cooking destroy valuable vitamins and minerals needed to keep your body healthy. Plenty of vitamins and minerals are present in natural foods like wholemeal bread and pasta, brown rice and other whole grains, as well as beans, pulses, nuts, fresh fruit and vegetables.

Meat and dairy produce. You don't need to cut meat from your diet – unless you want to! – but it is wise to limit your intake to one or two meals a week. This way you will be reducing your intake of saturated fats, but not going without meat altogether. Many people object to the way livestock is reared in inhumane conditions. One alternative is to choose produce that has been reared in organic and free-range conditions. We always use free-range eggs, for instance.

Organic food. Good health and good food start in the soil. If soil is deficient then so is the food grown in it. Deficient crops don't grow properly and are prone to disease and pest attacks. The farming industry's answer is to add pesticides, chemicals and nitrogenous fertilizers to kill disease. The result is food full of harmful residue. Also foods are sprayed with chemicals so that they stay fresh longer in shops. Some of the vegetables we buy have been sprayed up to 47 times! Always wash any vegetables well, and try to grow your own or buy organically-grown produce when possible.

PLANNING YOUR HEALTHY DIET

Breakfast. People often say they can't face breakfast, but you should try. A good breakfast gives a good start to the day and avoids the eleven o'clock slump that has you reaching for the dreaded doughnut. Muesli is probably the most valuable breakfast food but others are fresh fruit, porridge (use skimmed milk to keep fat intake down), natural yoghurt, wholemeal toast with honey or sugar-free jam, poached or boiled free-range egg, or compote of dried fruit.

To drink, have fresh orange juice, herbal tea (there are many, so experiment until you find one you like), decaffeinated coffee or mineral water.

Lunch. Our favourite lunch-time snack is home-made soup with wholemeal bread. Purée lightly cooked vegetables with stock – nothing could be simpler – or use pulses, like lentils or split peas.

Try and have a good helping of salad as well (or have it on its own). Make sure it contains a wide selection of leaf and root vegetables and sprouted seeds and/or fruit.

Evening meal. Make your main meal a protein one. Choose from lean meat, fish, poultry, free-range eggs, cheese or a combination of plant foods, nuts, grains or pulses. Serve your meal with a raw vegetable salad or lightly steamed vegetables. Include leafy green vegetables.

Finish with fresh fruit, yoghurt or a small amount of low-fat cheese.

Drinks for lunch and dinner. Try mineral water (check the salt content – Perrier is quite high, and Evian or Volvic are good), a coffee substitute, fresh fruit or vegetable juices (try making your own, it's worth investing in a juicer). If drinking alcohol, restrict yourself to two glasses of dry white wine daily and avoid spirits, or have the equivalent in real ale or dry cider.

GUIDELINES FOR HEALTHY EATING

Empty your larder of all packets and cans of processed and additive-laden foods to avoid temptation. Don't give them to your friends – rubbish belongs in one place only.

1 Replace all refined and processed foods by 100 per cent live whole foods. Especially avoid white flour products.

2 Replace all white, demerara and Barbados sugar with molasses and molasses sugar when cooking, and with organic unheated honey when not cooking. All sugars should be used infrequently and in small amounts.

3 Replace table, cooking and sea salt by kelp and occasionally 'Biosalt' (biochemically balanced mineral salt compound).

4 Replace tea, coffee and cocoa by nutritious cereal drinks, unsweetened fruit juices, unsalted vegetable juices and herb teas.

5 If you eat meat, buy naturally reared animals. If in doubt buy fish, game and free-range poultry. Vitamin K is destroyed by freezing so buy liver fresh, not frozen.

6 Do not overcook meat.

7 If vegetarian, then obtain protein from sprouted seeds, grains and legumes, avocado pears, nuts, free-range eggs, brewers' yeast, soya products, yoghurt and green vegetables.

8 Replace butter and saturated heated fats and margarines with unheated polyunsaturated margarines and cold pressed vegetable oils such as sunflower, safflower and olive.

9 Replace chocolate with carob powder.

10 Replace baking powder, cream of tartar and bicarbonate of soda with free-range eggs, fresh lemon juice and plenty of fresh air obtained by sufficient beating or whisking.

11 When cooking vegetables remember the following principles. Eat the flowers – broccoli, cauliflower and purple sprouting broccoli etc. – raw whenever possible; eat the stems and leaves very lightly cooked; and eat the roots cooked a little more (except carrots, which should always be eaten raw). Cook potatoes in their skins.

12 Eat the leaves of roots – of beetroot, turnip and carrot etc. – in a salad or lightly cooked. Eat the outer green leaves of vegetables.

13 Eat fruits and vegetables as fresh as possible to obtain the maximum nutritional value. If stored, keep in a cool dark place, and leave the roots on lettuces, cabbages etc.

14 Replace food grown by artificial fertilizers by food grown organically or bio-dynamically.

15 Wash all fresh fruit and vegetables if you are doubtful of their origin to remove any possible chemical sprays. Wash all dried fruit to remove possible sulphur dioxide, mineral oils and grit.

16 Avoid soaking fresh fruit and vegetables in water – soluble vitamins will suffer. Avoid cooking wherever possible as this will reduce the vitamin, mineral and enzyme content of the food. Cook vegetables in the smallest amount of water or in no water at all. Err on the undercooked rather than the overcooked side.

17 Avoid cooking at temperatures above 100°C (212°F). Magnesium, vitamins C and E, some other vitamins and minerals and all enzymes can be destroyed (nutritionally) by heat. The enzymes begin to be destroyed at temperatures as low as 40°C (104°F). To offset these deficiencies in our cooked food, we must obtain them from raw food.

18 Ideally take two-thirds raw food to one-third cooked. Consume some raw food at every cooked meal.

19 Eat all herbs raw for the full mineral and vitamin content. When adding them to hot food, add them at the end of the cooking.

20 Use oil and lemon juice to prevent oxidation of shredded or

diced raw vegetables and green salad. Use lemon or orange juice for freshly cut fruit. Take fresh fruit and a fresh green salad daily.

21 Grow sprouts from seeds, grains and legumes all the year round – this does not require a garden. Grow as much food as you can following organic principles.

22 Never cook with aluminium pans. Use stainless steel or iron utensils.

23 Remove the pepper and salt cruet and replace by three salt shakers, one filled with paprika, one with kelp powder and the other with brewers' yeast.

24 Avoid cigarettes, spirits and drugs.

25 Have available seeds, nuts and dried fruits if a meal has been missed or for the children when they come home from school. Sunflower seeds are tasty and very nutritious.

26 Avoid rich and concentrated desserts and cakes, even when made of nutritious ingredients, except when entertaining.

27 Avoid snacks between meals. This indicates that the quality of main meals is not nutritionally adequate. Sugar-containing snacks are likely to greatly increase the risk of tooth decay.

28 Avoid eating when tired, emotionally upset or when in a hurry. The digestive processes will be impaired.

29 Avoid drinking with meals that are based on sound nutrition. Drink an hour before a meal or two hours afterwards to avoid diluting the digestive juices. The one exception to the rule is if you ever have the misfortune to get landed with an over-salted or over-sugared meal; if you eat it, then to drink with the meal is your only salvation.

30 Only drink when you are thirsty. On a diet based on sound nutrition you will find that very little drinking will be necessary. Most of the food you will be eating will contain a large percentage of water.

31 Do not eat too late in the evening. One should breakfast like a king, lunch like a prince and sup like a pauper – and the latter should be as early as possible to allow digestion to take place before sleep.

32 When feeling unwell, cold or shivery, or when suffering from a sore throat, avoid eating all foods except fresh fruits and vegetables containing an abundance of Vitamin C.

33 Thoroughly chew your food so that it is a tasteless pulp which can melt away and does not have to be consciously swallowed. This carries out the first stage of digestion in the mouth, and prepares the rest of the digestive system and body to absorb the nutrients more efficiently.

34 Remember that it is not the *amount* that we eat, but the amount that we *assimilate* that nourishes.

Never put off till tomorrow what you can do today. It may be too late, especially where your health is concerned.

CHAPTER ELEVEN

What the Future May Hold

Today's unorthodoxy is tomorrow's convention! Some of the therapies I will discuss below may be regarded by some as unorthodox. I believe that by increasing our knowledge and broadening our outlook, some of the orthodox treatments of today will appear crude, and in most cases ineffectual, compared with what the future may bring. So where does dentistry go from here? At present the science has progressed on all fronts: treatment and patient comfort have become more 'civilized'; dental techniques and equipment have increasingly high standards; new materials are constantly being introduced with improved qualities; and the education at both undergraduate and postgraduate levels is reaching new heights in excellence. The training of dentists in the UK is undoubtedly amongst the best in the world.

Using the Body's Energy to Diagnose Disease

As any practitioner knows, diagnosis is fundamental to any cure. You cannot treat a disease or malfunction of the body without knowing the cause. When treating disease and malfunctions of the body, medical science up to now has concentrated to a large degree on biochemistry. This has proved invaluable in the diagnosis, treatment, and in some cases the total eradication of disease, of smallpox, diphtheria, TB, and polio, for instance. And since the discovery of penicillin, vaccines and disinfectants, many life-threatening infections and diseases of the past are now regarded as relatively minor. However, although the advantages of drugs such as antibiotics, steroids and pain-killers are many, it is often said that these medications are treating the *effects* of disease and ill-health rather than the *cause*, and that the medical profession has become too reliant upon them. We should look, therefore, at many other disciplines, and see what they offer – perhaps even learn from them.

ENERGIES

Few diagnostic advances have been made in the field of biophysics – the way in which the human body works and responds to various forms of energy. Those likely to affect our bodies are electricity, magnetism, gravitation and nuclear energy. Some are known already to be harmful – the radiation from an atomic bomb or over-exposure to X-rays, for instance – but some of our other 'destructive' research could be channelled *con*structively. Much research is being carried out into using high-energy lasers as a weapon in the Star Wars program. However, low-energy 'cold lasers' are being used to accelerate wound healing, and some dentists claim that these energies can calm down the inflammation of a painful tooth.

Another form of energy which is harmful in large doses is sunlight; a small amount, however, that which we take in during a British summer, helps the body utilize calcium by converting one form of Vitamin D into a form more useful to the body. And calcium which, as we know, is an important mineral dentally, can also be affected by electricity and magnetism. Astronauts were found to lose calcium from their bones when spending long periods in space. Scientists came to the obvious conclusion that being weightless, their bones and muscles did not need to work so hard thus allowing the bones to become 'softer'. Later research showed that this change in calcium metabolism was found to be connected with the weaker magnetic field found in space than that on the surface of the earth.

If anyone doubts that these energies can affect their mental approach to things, one only needs to experience the oppressive feeling before a thunderstorm. At this time there is a very high concentration of positive ions in the atmosphere: immediately after the storm the situation is reversed, when there is a high concentration of negative ions with the accompanying feeling of well-being. Many dentists utilize this phenomenon by installing ionizers in their surgeries. They often report that both themselves and their patients feel less tense, and that their surgery 'atmosphere' is improved.

ACUPUNCTURE AND RELATED THERAPIES

At present physicians of all disciplines take physical measurements of the body's energy to detect disease and malfunctions. Taking the pulse, measuring blood pressure and tapping the knee for nerve reflexes are simple tests with which we are all familiar. The heart scan (ECG), brain scan (EEG), X-rays and ultrasound are also valuable tools in diagnosis. Electro-diagnosis is a recent method of measuring energy imbalances in the body. It has been found that each body organ produces or consumes energy, and that health is an energetic equilibrium which can be influenced through the acupuncture points. Electronic instruments have been designed to measure the slightest energy variations in these points, and the technique is being researched and used in medical practices in countries such as the USA, Germany and France. (In Great Britain there is a growing interest – but we lag behind.)

There are few health professionals who do *not* accept that, used correctly, acupuncture can be an effective medical 'tool'. Many have tried to explain the workings of acupuncture using the body's normal nervous pathways; the theory being that by stimulating nerves from one part of the body, the brain does not perceive pain from another. Unfortunately, life is not so simple and the latest research indicates that the older Chinese principle appears more plausible. This is that the basic life energy, Ch'i (pronounced Chee), is present in every living creature and that it circulates along specific pathways in the body called meridians, or channels of energy flow (CEF). These meridians may follow the normal nervous pathways, but often do not: some meridians follow the lymphatic system whilst others have been charted which do not correspond to any known biological network.

There are areas of the body where the skin exhibits a lower electrical resistance (over 4,000 points have been found), and these represent acupuncture points. As long as Ch'i flows freely through the meridians, health is maintained. When the flow of energy is blocked, for any reason, there is disruption of health resulting in pain and disease. By stimulating appropriate

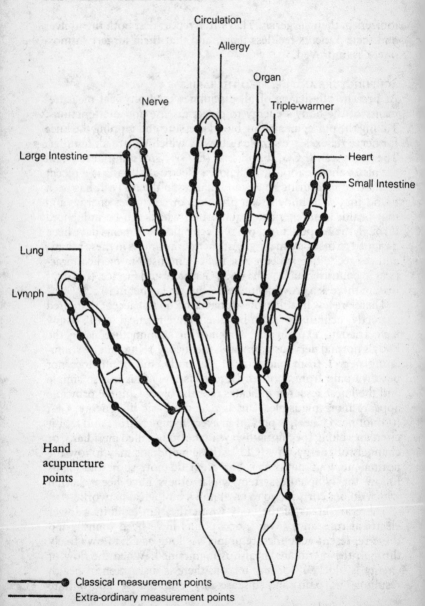

Circulation

Allergy

Organ

Triple-warmer

Nerve

Large Intestine

Heart

Small Intestine

Lung

Lymph

Hand
acupuncture
points

●——— Classical measurement points

——— Extra-ordinary measurement points

acupuncture points the blocked energy is released and health is restored. The hands, feet and ears are very important areas of the body for acupuncture diagnosis and treatment.

Practitioners using the above techniques are truly holistic. They are looking at the interaction of individual organs or systems within the whole body. The mouth and teeth, for instance, appear to have a very significant effect on other parts of the body. Many practitioners of differing specialities have reported that, when tracing the cause of their patient's malaise, the teeth and jaws appear to be implicated. Thus I am obliged to say that we, as dentists, may not yet fully comprehend the significance of dental disease and its effects on the rest of the body's well-being. Already, when discussing the TMJ syndrome, the effects of malfunction have been shown to be widespread. What may be the effect of gum disease, of tooth decay and root abscesses on the whole body?

From personal observation, I have noticed that after treatments to remove foci of infection from the mouth, patients often feel generally much better, both physically and mentally. Researchers and practitioners of acupuncture have found that disturbances of the teeth and jaws can affect their diagnosing and treatment, and regard the health of the mouth as important. Although acupuncture has been practised for thousands of years, scientists are still making advances in understanding the mechanism of how and why it works. In that process, the knowledge of how the body works is also unfolding a little more.

Electro-therapy. Electronic instruments designed to vary the strength and frequency of the electronic pulses they emit are already being used to control and minimize pain. These instruments incorporate certain acupuncture principles and techniques. Instead of needling, the acupuncture points are treated electrically. As the damaged tissue areas receive the correct flow of electrical energies the circulation improves and the normal healing process is accelerated. This technique can be used for injuries such as surgical wounds, fractures, bruises and sprains, as well as arthritis, painful trigger zones and diseased tissue. In many professional sports such as football, basketball, and rugby, a team physician with the skills to use electronic therapy is employed.

When correctly used, electro-therapy can immediately reduce

pain, which is obviously gratifying to the patient, and this could be of considerable use in dentistry. Acute dental pain can be the most severe a person is likely to suffer and any effective technique to give immediate relief must be welcome. Electro-acupuncture could be used to numb the jaw so that fillings may be carried out, or so that a tooth could be extracted painlessly. This may be of special value to patients who suffer multiple allergies and for whom the use of drugs to induce anaesthesia would be inadvisable. There are also an increasing number of people who disagree with any form of drug therapy – and indeed many who are pathologically frightened of needles. Electro-therapy could be offered as an alternative.

I am certain that the future of acupuncture is exciting – both as a means of diagnosis and treatment – and that it will become a vital instrument in the hands of our next generation of dentists as well as doctors.

APPLIED KINESIOLOGY (AK)
AK is a system of dealing with functional health disturbances, and it uses the patient's body as a laboratory of investigation. Unlike pathology – the state of tissue alteration to be studied under a microscope – AK deals largely with functional processes such as the movement and strength of muscles and their relationship with stress, and is a totally new concept. It began about twenty years ago, and had its origins in the chiropractic profession. AK is rapidly gaining credence all over the world, however, and many dentists and physicians of all disciplines are using it, to a lesser or greater degree, in their practices. I believe that this is a very important discovery, although still in its developmental stages, because of the vast usages AK may have to the holistic practitioner. The following descriptions may appear like voodoo, but much work and research has been carried out and the claims of the protagonists appear to have been verified. Having seen many demonstrations and having used simple techniques myself, all I can say is that some of the applications of AK appear quite mind-boggling!

Diagnostic or muscle testing is perhaps the most remarkable part of the discovery of AK. The principle – which appears to hold true – is that the body will 'tell' the practitioner what is wrong if it is 'asked'. This may sound strange, and a few examples are in order. A patient with a history of allergies is asked to put out an arm sideways so that the arm is parallel to the ground. The practitioner will then lay one hand on the patient's shoulder and rest two fingers on the patient's wrist. The patient will then be asked to resist the practitioner's attempt to push down the arm. Let's say, for example, that the practitioner could not lower the arm, or could only do so with a great deal of force: the patient tested strong. (The amount of force needed to overcome the patient's arm strength could, of course, be measured with a spring balance – a method perhaps favoured by the more scientific.) After this initial strength test, the practitioner may then place a minute amount of a certain food on, or under, the patient's tongue (the type of food kept secret from the patient), and the test repeated. This time the patient appears to have very little strength and the slightest pressure makes the arm go down. The patient has tested weak. The practitioner, in this example an allergist, may then conclude that the food substance does not agree with the patient.

One might say that the patient 'thought' weak, or that many other variables influenced the result. But researchers using placebos and blind and double-blind research techniques, have obtained results that appear remarkably consistent. Anyone can try this test with foods like white sugar or salt and, more interestingly, with drugs like pain-killers and tranquillizers. Many will be surprised how weak they test, especially on the latter, which they may be using regularly. Muscle testing is not a game. Health is far too important, and I stress that those who specialize in AK need to undergo a great deal of training and experience. A little knowledge can be a bad thing.

It is unclear why a weakness occurs when there is an imbalance in the body. It is not just biochemical upsets as described above that can cause a drop in strength, but all forms of stress. From a holistic standpoint the situation is clear: stress, no matter how small, be it chemical, physical or emotional, will affect the whole body. Dentists have a particular interest in AK, for if the above muscle-testing procedure is repeated on a patient with suspected TMJ syndrome, a quick test may tell the practitioner that at least part of the problem lies in the jaw. The patient may test strong with the mouth open and weak with the teeth clenched. Although not conclusive, any aid to verify a diagnosis must be welcomed. As in a chiropractic clinic, the holistic dentist may find kinesiological testing useful in getting information about structural imbalances in the whole body. And, as nutrition is profoundly important to the dentist, AK can be used to check a patient's dietary regime, and can even verify how much of a given supplement or drug is required to improve health.

I am sure that much of the mystique which surrounds some aspects of AK will disappear as investigations continue. At present it is like twentieth-century practitioners using twenty-first-century techniques. To quote George J. Goodheart, one of the founders of this new science, 'The name of the game is to get people better. The body heals itself in a sure, sensible, practical, reasonable and observable manner. The healer within can be approached from without.' And at least five years ago, Dr Gelb, a TMJ specialist, said that he predicted that medical and dental specialists will use applied kinesiological testing to make more accurate diagnosis and provide better treatment. I believe this is already slowly happening.

HOMOEOPATHY

Homoeopathy is both a method of treatment and a medical philosophy. It is practised throughout the world, and in France all pharmacies are required by law to give homoeopathic prescriptions as well as prescriptions for drugs from conventional doctors. A German physician, Samuel Hahnemann, developed the medical system of homoeopathy in the late eighteenth century, but physicians have known and used the fundamental principles for over 2,000 years.

If asked, most homoeopaths would say that their medicines are founded on three basic principles:

1 A medicine which in large doses produces the symptoms of a disease will, in small doses, cure that disease.

2 By extreme dilution, the medicine's curative properties are enhanced, and all the poisonous or undesirable side-effects are lost.

3 Homoeopathic medicines are prescribed individually by the

study of the whole person, according to basic temperament and responses.

Homoeopathic dosages treat and cure in a gentle and profound manner by using the natural defence mechanisms of the body – similar in principle to vaccinations.

Many conventionally trained doctors also practise homoeopathy. The effectiveness of the treatment relies as much upon the homoeopathic practitioner as upon the medicine prescribed. Homoeopathy has both restricted and broad uses and enables the practitioner to carry out preventive treatment in fields where conventional therapy is totally unsuitable. In dentistry, there are many areas in which homoeopathy may help. Camilla 6 can be used to relieve the traumas of teething. Wound healing and pain relief after dental extractions, deep scaling or surgery could be other possibilities, and arnica may be prescribed. Ulcerated gums, a metallic taste in the mouth and bad breath could possibly be helped by merc. sol. Even the fear of attending the dentist may be reduced by argent nit. Many will say that the amount of the 'medicine' is so small that any beneficial effect is 'in the mind'. If this is the case, it seems surprising that even animals like horses, dogs and cats can make remarkable recoveries from illness following homoeopathic treatment.

My knowledge of homoeopathy is comparatively limited, but many of my patients use these remedies to great effect. Again, more research and experience is needed to place homoeopathy in the mainstream of medicine, but I feel that it will undeniably be the medicine of the future.

Dental Breakthroughs

So far I have briefly described some new exciting concepts which have far-reaching applications for the whole body as well as for the dental tissues. But there are areas of dental research which, if 'breakthroughs' occur, could mean the end of tooth decay and the lessening of gum disease. I feel the most promising are in the areas of vaccine and enzymes.

Take the simple formula that can be applied to dental disease:

Bacteria + saliva = plaque
Plaque + sugar = tooth decay

Should we remove any one of the components of the formula then the disease process will be prevented. Plaque can be removed from the formula by good oral hygiene as previously discussed, and sugar can be removed by diet modification: these are both simple and natural ways of arresting the disease process. However, there are many people who still smoke, although they know its harmful effects, and there are perhaps equally as many who do not brush their teeth effectively or who will never give up consuming large amounts of sugar.

VACCINE

If a vaccine could be developed that would change the oral flora (the bacteria that live in the mouth) in such a way that the species of bacteria which have been thought to produce acid or have been implicated in the disease process, are effectively removed, then plaque may not form, or if it does, no acid will be produced when sugar is added. Research into such a vaccine is not new, and as yet no breakthrough has been announced. As with all biochemical discoveries, even if the product works in the part of the body it is designed to affect, one must always question possible side-effects. As described before, the reactions and dynamics taking place in the mouth are multiple and complex, but if a *completely* safe vaccine were to be discovered, then the discoverer would have the distinct honour of curing 'the most common disease in the world'.

ENZYMES

Many biochemists and dental researchers are looking at another part of the dental disease equation, the saliva. Saliva has multiple protective qualities (see Chapter Four), but of particular interest to scientists are the enzymes that affect the oral bacteria. Salivary enzymes with names like Lactoperoxidase, Thiocynate, Lactofferine, and Lysozyme, to name but a few, can alter the way bacteria grow, reproduce and exist. By increasing the amount of some of these enzymes (nature's antibiotics) artificially, plaque growth can be inhibited or the adverse effects of plaque altered.

Several toothpastes are now 'enzymic', and contain one or more enzyme systems designed to produce and slow down the development of plaque. The results from research trials do appear to show that these toothpastes are effective. Having taken a very cautious attitude in recommending enzymic toothpaste to my patients, I am receiving many reports confirming that, in conjunction with regular oral hygiene, the rate of development of plaque appears to be slower. As with any new product, adverse reactions must be carefully monitored. The effectiveness of such a system relies, unfortunately, upon the assumption that teeth will be regularly brushed with these toothpastes but, looking at overall sales figures for the country, this does not appear to be the case.

Drill-less Dentistry!

When a tooth cavity is prepared for a filling there are two main objectives: to remove all diseased tissue, and to shape the cavity to retain the filling effectively and prevent any further disease or breakdown of the surrounding tooth structure. To achieve the above, the most widely used instrument is the drill – either the whining high-speed air rotor, or the slower (bumpy) drill. Cavity preparation may soon be accomplished without the use of the drill. Research is being carried out into using solutions capable of dissolving the diseased or decayed part of the tooth without damaging the harder and sounder parts. Besides the advantages of no drilling, this procedure would be less painful, making the need for anaesthetics – 'the needle' – less likely. But cavities in teeth are not always the ideal shape for filling, and, after having dissolved away our tooth decay, how then can we overcome problems of retaining the filling? Modern techniques may have the answer. Instead of cutting a lock to key the filling into the tooth, the retention for the filling can be obtained by microscopic holes etched into the surface of the cavity. The currently used composite filling can then be applied. The only drilling that may be required will be to shape and polish the surface.

Aims of the Future

The first priority of any healing profession must be to eliminate disease and the suffering therefrom. I believe tooth decay and gum disease can be completely eradicated, and it is towards this aim that we must direct our researches. The other priority is to improve both the function and the cosmetic appearance of teeth and jaws to the best possible benefit of our patients: this gives not only the potent psychological benefit of a pleasing appearance, but also a general well-being of the body as a whole.

To achieve all this, I believe certain changes are needed in the dental practitioner's philosophy, and I classify them below.

1 Dentists must follow a multi-disciplinarian and holistic approach. We must integrate both practically and theoretically with all the other health professions, such as medical doctors, scientists, biochemists, bio-engineers, nutritionists, osteopaths, applied kinesiologists and other recognized practitioners.

2 Dentists must institute a preventative programme that will start even before conception and will continue throughout life. The investment in time and money for such a programme will pay handsome dividends in terms of sparing pain, discomfort, loss of time and, of course, money.

3 Given that we are not in an ideal world, unfortunately, I predict that dentists will still be carrying out unnecessary treatment for at least the foreseeable future. Techniques need to be developed to make the treatment of dental disease completely painless, effective and long-lasting, and to improve the tools we need for diagnosis and treatment.

Selected Bibliography

John Besford, *Good Mouthkeeping*, Debeli Press, 1980

Geoffrey Cannon and Caroline Walker, *The Food Scandal*, Century, 1985

R. A. Cawson, *Essentials of Dental Surgery and Pathology*, Churchill Livingstone, 1978

Cooper Products, *Current Aspects of Dental Health*, 1983

Cowell and Sheihan, *Promoting Dental Health*, King Edwards Hospital Fund, Pitman Books, 1981

Dr C. Curtis Shears, *Nutritional Science and Health Education*, Castle Press, 1974

John Forrest, *The Good Teeth Guide*, Granada, 1981

Doris Grant, *Fluoridation and the Forgotten Issue*, National Anti-Fluoridation Campaign

Harold Gelb and Paula M. Siegel, *Killing Pain Without Prescription*, Thorsons, 1983

Miranda Hall, *Feeding Your Children*, Piatkus Books, 1984

Maurice Hansson, *E for Additives*, Thorsons, 1985

Walter Hoffman-Anthelm, *History of Dentistry*, Quintessence Publishing Co., 1981

G. Neil Jenkins, *The Physiology and Biochemistry of the Mouth*, Blackwell Scientific Publications, 1978

Dr Hugh Jolly, *The Book of Child Care*, Sphere, 1981

Leslie and Susannah Kenton, *Raw Energy*, Century, 1984

Penelope Leach, *Baby and Child*, Penguin, 1982

Lilian Lindsay, *A Short History of Dentistry*, John Bale, Sons, and Danielsson Ltd, 1933

Shklar McCarthy, *The Oral Manifestations of Systemic Disease*, Butterworths, 1976

J. D. Manson, *Periodontics*, Henry Kimpton, 1966

Dr Weston Price, *Nutrition and Physical Degeneration*, Price-Pottenger Foundation, 1970

Herman Prinz, *Dental Chronology*, Henry Kimpton, 1945

Patricia M. Randolph and Carol I. Dennison, *Diet, Nutrition and Dentistry*, The C. V. Mosby Company, 1981

Elizabeth Shears, *Why Do We Eat?*, Mulberry Press, 1976

Dr Sheldon B. Sidney, *Ignore Your Teeth and They'll Go Away*, Devida Publications, 1982

Drs Penny and Andrew Stanway, *Breast is Best*, Pan, 1978

G. C. Van Beek, *Dental Morphology*, Wright Publishing Co., 1983

John Woodforde, *The Strange Story of False Teeth*, Tandem, 1968

Professor John Yudkin, *Pure, White and Deadly*, Davis-Poynter Ltd, 1972

Sam Ziff, *The Toxic Time-Bomb*, Aurora Press, 1984

Index

Page numbers in *italic* refer to the illustrations